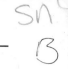

Overcoming Depression and Low Mood

A five areas approach

Overcoming Depression and Low Mood

A five areas approach

Second edition

Dr Chris Williams MBChB BSc MMedSc MD FRCPsych

Senior Lecturer and Honorary Consultant Psychiatrist
Section of Psychological Medicine
University of Glasgow Medical School
Glasgow, UK

A five areas approach
Helping you to help yourself
www.livinglifetothefull.com

Hodder Arnold

A MEMBER OF THE HODDER HEADLINE GROUP

First published in Great Britain in 2001 by Arnold
Revised 2002
This second edition published in 2006 by
Hodder Arnold, an imprint of Hodder Education and a member of the Hodder Headline Group,
338 Euston Road, London NW1 3BH

http://www.hoddereducation.com

Distributed in the United States of America by
Oxford University Press Inc.,
198 Madison Avenue, New York NY10016
Oxford is a registered trademark of Oxford University Press

British Library Cataloguing in Publication Data
A catalogue record for this book is available from the British Library

Library of Congress Cataloging-in-Publication Data
A catalog record for this book is available from the Library of Congress

ISBN 978 0 340 90586 9

2 3 4 5 6 7 8 9 10

Commissioning Editor: Clare Christian/Philip Shaw
Project Editor: Clare Patterson
Production Controller: Karen Tate
Cover Designer: Nichola Smith
Cartoon illustrations: Keith Chan

Typeset in 11 on 15 pt Sabon by Phoenix Photosetting, Chatham, Kent
Printed and bound in Great Britain by CPI Bath

What do you think about this book? Or any other Hodder Arnold title?
Please send your comments to www.hoddereducation.com

New ways of accessing the workbooks
Buying the book in bulk: bulk copies of the book are available at discounted rates direct from the publisher.

5–30 copies: 25%
31–50 copies: 30%
51–100 copies: 40%
101–200 copies: 45%
200+ copies: 50%

To take advantage of these reduced rates please contact Jane MacRae, Sales Development Manager, Hodder Headline, 338 Euston Road, London NW1 3BH. Tel +44 (0)20 7873 6146. Email janemacrae@hodder.co.uk

Details of other ways of delivering the course are available at www.livinglifetothefull.com and www.fiveareas.com

Contents

Foreword: a user's viewpoint

Depression Alliance Scotland is the leading national charity working to provide information and support for people affected by depression in Scotland. The charity supports principles of self-management and self-help in improving the understanding of depression and in enabling greater coping mechanisms and recovery in relation to the illness. It is of great significance to our work that the recent National Institute for Clinical Excellence (NICE) guideline for England recommends that for mild and moderate depression, psychological treatments focused specifically on depression, such as problem-solving therapy and cognitive behaviour therapy (CBT), can be as effective as drug treatments and should be offered as treatment options. The guideline on depression also states that 'antidepressants are not recommended for the initial treatment of mild depression' and advises practitioners to 'inform patients, families and carers about self-help and support groups, and encourage them to participate where appropriate'. Self-help approaches such as this set of workbooks provide additional non-pharmacological options in the management of the illness.

We know from people who use our services that many people with depression struggle to seek help or access the appropriate support they need. Common concerns reported include issues such as stigma and social isolation, stress and anxiety, loss, bereavement, physical health problems, relationship problems, financial difficulties and employment issues, problems with professionals, concerns about medication, and a general lack of support and available treatment options. Along with colleagues in Depression Alliance Scotland, I have attended training courses in using the five areas style of working and find the materials a valuable and timely contribution to tackling depression.

I find this series of supported self-help workbooks to be an excellent and timely resource. The workbooks are extremely informative, well written and well developed, and are a worthy addition to the current self-help resources on offer. The book is for use by people experiencing clinical depression as well as for people with low mood. It is divided into clear topical workbooks and covers many of the common concerns that people with depression can face. The book offers clear information about depression and the key contributory factors. It also recognises the sheer awfulness of depression and aims to help readers make changes at a pace that is appropriate for them. The workbooks offer practical interventions and adopt a stage-by-stage approach through each section to support the reader in recognising the potential to make positive changes where relevant.

A helpful addition is a section for friends and relatives of people experiencing depression, which aims to help anyone in this position to offer effective support to someone experiencing depression and to understand more about the illness.

In summary, the workbooks are user-friendly and throughout demonstrate respect for the individual nature of depression and how it affects people. Depression Alliance Scotland sees the book as having the potential to increase a person's confidence in their own ability to make changes and move forward in their life. As an organisation, we are beginning to introduce educational sessions using the workbook content into our group meetings, and we also have started a new life-skills course that is delivered in further education colleges and is based on these workbooks. This joint project between ourselves and the NHS has been well received and, we trust, will develop further.

Ilena Day
National Coordinator, Depression Alliance Scotland

Foreword: a general practitioner's viewpoint

As a general practitioner, I have a long-standing interest in depression, due to both the distress that it causes to my patients and the major impact that it has upon providing general medical care. A quarter of all consultations in general practice are concerned with mental health, and 90% of people with such problems are helped by their general practitioner without referral to specialists. Not only is depression an important and life-threatening illness, but it is also often combined with chronic physical disease, further increasing the person's distress.

The lowering of mood that occurs in depression can easily make the treatments offered appear unattractive or overwhelming, further reducing hope of improvement. Despite its seriousness, however, depression is a highly treatable condition and there is an increasing recognition of when and how to introduce the most appropriate therapies.

Often, depression responds well to exercise programmes or to drug treatments, and the effectiveness of combining physical and psychological treatments is now well recognised. Of the psychological treatments available, cognitive behaviour therapy (CBT) is proven to be effective both at improving the rate of recovery from an acute episode of depression and, importantly, in greatly reducing the risk of recurrence of a further episode. At present, however, there is a significant shortage of therapists trained to deliver CBT and other forms of psychological treatment to those who might benefit.

Unfortunately, unlike drug treatments, the production lines of CBT cannot be speeded up easily and it takes considerable time and training to produce specialist therapists able to provide skilled individual treatment to patients. My interest in depression and other mental health problems led me to train as a cognitive behaviour therapist. Despite my own training, however, it is not possible for me to provide 'full' CBT to more than a small proportion of my patients who might otherwise benefit.

Is there an answer to this dilemma? One of the most promising solutions to the problem has been the development of self-help books and other materials that can provide much of the structure, information and teaching of the key skills involved in CBT. The first edition of this book was one such self-help book and uses a user-friendly form of CBT, the *five areas model* developed by Dr Chris Williams and colleagues.

The five areas model is a great aid in helping to make sense of many of the symptoms of depression, and other common problems often faced in life. This includes the combination of physical sensations, emotional distress, difficult social and other circumstances, unhelpful thinking patterns and behaviours that so often make up distress.

The package consists of manageable workbooks, each designed to be read over one or two weeks, with the opportunity for self-review between workbooks. The workbooks can also be supported by a trusted family member or friend as well as healthcare practitioners. The workbooks place great emphasis on a thorough learning of the basic principles of CBT, such as recognising the links between thoughts, feelings and behaviour, before moving on to more involved and sophisticated techniques, such as how to identify and challenge extreme and unhelpful thinking. The individual workbooks of *Overcoming Depression and Low Mood* can enable patients and those supporting them to see and understand these interacting patterns much more clearly. It is the teaching of these basic principles that can so easily be overlooked, even by an experienced therapist. The pacing, reinforcement and repetition are all highly appropriate for patients who may be far from well and with considerable impairment of both concentration and memory.

This new edition has been designed to be even more user-friendly, enabling patients to do the vast majority of the work of CBT in their own time. This, then, can make it easier for additional and realistic support to be provided by a health professional, who might be a nurse, doctor or other health worker within a practice team.

The self-help approach provided by *Overcoming Depression and Low Mood* is very much in line with recent guidelines, which strongly encourage self-help approaches such as this. The course can both be empowering and also make a real difference in the lives of those who use it. From a combination of research evidence and my own clinical experience, there is now little doubt that *Overcoming Depression and Low Mood* provides one extremely helpful solution.

In summary, I believe that *Overcoming Depression and Low Mood* has already proved to be a very valuable addition to our therapeutic resources and has made a real impact upon the problem of how to treat depression in general practice. By providing patients with this truly powerful and useable tool, it will empower and improve the quality of their lives and enable health professionals to use their own skills in increasingly effective and appropriate ways. Once again, I look forward to using it in my own practice.

Dr Steve Williams, MRCP, MRCGP
General Practitioner, the Garth Surgery, Guisborough, Cleveland

Foreword: an expert cognitive behavioural therapist's viewpoint

This second edition of *Overcoming Depression and Low Mood* has all the hallmarks of the excellent first edition. It presents the practical strategies of an empirically validated psychological treatment for depression as a user-friendly resource. The treatment package uses the principles and practices of cognitive behaviour therapy (CBT), which are presented as a series of structured self-help workbooks that can be used individually in stand-alone format or in combination as a step-wise approach to tackling depression. The workbooks are written for use by individuals looking for help to manage their low mood and depression. It will also prove helpful for healthcare practitioners seeking a useful tool for working with patients who are experiencing a depressive episode.

The clear and easy-to-follow format, with a highly accessible reading age, means the workbooks can also be utilised in a broad range of service settings, including primary and secondary care and non-health settings such as public libraries and self-help programmes within the voluntary sector. The package lends itself well as a key resource for mental health nurses in a variety of settings, including community mental health teams, in-patient services, day hospital settings and primary care. Health visitors and practice nurses will also find the workbooks useful, and the book will be invaluable to GPs, psychiatrists and clinical psychologists.

This updated version is true to the original format, presenting a pragmatic, problem-solving approach aimed at equipping the user with a range of strategies that facilitate effective mood management using core CBT skills. This includes activity scheduling and graded task assignment, identifying and modifying unhelpful automatic thoughts, and basic problem-solving skills – all done without using jargon.

In the spirit of evidence-based practice, as new developments in the CBT field for treating depression have emerged and with the author's experience of using the workbooks in a variety of clinical and non-clinical settings, this second edition has been revised to improve accessibility and extend the scope of each workbook. This has given *Overcoming Depression and Low Mood* added value in terms of its usefulness within a stepped care programme, ranging from self-help to assisted self-help and as part of more formalised individual and group-based treatments available for depression.

This self-help book comes highly recommended. It is sufficiently flexible to be integrated into a range of healthcare and non-healthcare settings. Its user-friendly format makes it an easy-to-use package that has the potential to increase accessibility to CBT for depression and improve the cost-effectiveness of services.

Anne Garland

Nurse Consultant in Psychological Therapies, Nottingham

Introduction

Welcome to *Overcoming Depression and Low Mood*. This fully revised and updated second edition is based on over five years' experience of work using this approach. At the same time, self-help approaches are being used increasingly within the National Health Service as one of a number of ways of overcoming problems of low mood and depression.

This book has developed out of a wide range of work that has focused on how best to support people using self-help materials delivered in all sorts of different ways. The aim is to help readers to help themselves by providing clearly described practical tools to help them make changes. The hope is that you will find encouragement and feel empowered to make changes yourself.

Who is the book for?

Many different people may be using this book. You may be using the resources for yourself, or perhaps you are a close friend or family member wanting to know more about depression and low mood. Many healthcare practitioners also use these workbooks to support the patients they work with. Our research and clinical practice have shown that the book can be used by people with problems ranging from mild distress through to more severe depression. The treatment approach involves reading the course workbooks and also working on problems. If your concentration, energy or motivation levels are far lower than usual and you find it very hard to keep your mind on things or to make changes, then now may not be the right time to use this course. Other approaches such as antidepressants may be more appropriate first, allowing you to come back to use the workbooks at a time when you are able to get the most from them. Likewise, if you find that you struggle to use the workbooks or you feel worse as you work through them, please discuss this with your doctor or healthcare practitioner.

How does the book work?

Have you ever had the experience of someone saying to you 'What you said last time really made a great difference' and yet you can't remember quite what you said? Perhaps something similar has happened to you when you have been mulling over a problem and a friend or relative has said something that really helped put things into perspective. This common experience indicates that providing the right information or question can make a real difference to how we feel. The concept of using sequences of effective questions and information is the basis of cognitive behaviour therapy (CBT), which has a proven effectiveness in the treatment of depression. As a practitioner, I have had a lot of experience both in clinical practice and in setting up and evaluating service delivery of CBT and CBT self-help. As a teacher, I have struggled to address the issues of how to engage people in learning and applying what they learn. This includes the challenge of how to explain things in a way that draws people in to talk about the things they want to learn. Finally, as a researcher, I have had the opportunity to be able to test out and evaluate these and related self-help materials and to refine the contents based on this research. I hope that the coming together of these three influences – clinical practice, teaching and research – adds to the course content.

What will you learn?

The course contains workbooks that address all the main problem areas affected during times of low mood. The workbooks will help you discover why you feel as you do and teach you key skills that you can use to improve things.

In reading these workbooks, you will:
- Discover why you feel as you do.
- Develop better problem-solving skills.

- Rebalance relationships by becoming more assertive.
- Become more active and rediscover the fun in life.
- Build helpful responses to life stresses.
- Discover how to sleep better.
- Learn how to change negative and undermining thinking.
- Stop reacting in ways that backfire.
- Make choices that boost a healthy lifestyle.
- Plan for the future in order to stay well.

A further workbook is aimed at the friends and relatives of those with low mood and depression and describes how best to offer support.

There is no right or wrong way to use the workbooks. Many people find it most helpful to read the first two workbooks in Part 1 (*Starting out* and *Understanding why I feel as I do*) to help gain an overview of the approach. This will also help you to decide which of the 'making changes' workbooks in Part 2 of the book you will read. You can use as many or as few workbooks in the course as you wish. A key to creating change in your life is using the workbooks and putting what you learn into practice.

A word of encouragement

No one is immune from depression. Depression and low mood are common and affect many people. They can affect each of us in all sorts of ways. Fortunately, it has now become clear that changing certain thoughts and behaviour patterns can have a significant impact on improving how we feel. The content of these workbooks is based upon the CBT approach. This has identified effective ways of tackling many of the common symptoms and problems faced when we feel low. Each workbook will teach you important information about how depression and low mood affect you. They also will help you learn some practical skills that you can use to bring about positive change. The workbooks aim to help you to regain a sense of control over how you feel.

Sometimes, making changes is easier said (or written) than done. All of us feel discouraged and overwhelmed from time to time. This is even more likely to occur in times of low mood. I want to really encourage you to try to make a commitment to use this course and to keep at it, even if you feel discouraged or stuck for a time. To do this, you will need to pace yourself by using a step-by-step approach. Bear in mind what your motivation and energy levels allow you to do, so you don't bite off more than you can chew. This will help you to get as much from the course as you can at the moment.

The workbook that follows – *Starting out* – gives some suggestions of how you can pace things and also some suggestions of what you can do if you are struggling.

Visual or reading problems: large print, Betsie reader and online audio-based versions of the materials are also available at www.livinglifetothefull.com.

Two new online resources have been written to also support users of the course:

- **For users of the book:** www.livinglifetothefull.com – helping you to help yourself. This completely free website supported by the Scottish Executive Health Department contains short talks that help you to build upon the course workbooks. In addition, handout resources, online relaxation tapes and a moderated discussion forum allow those using the book to swap ideas, hints and tips and offer and receive mutual support.

- **For healthcare practitioners:** www.fiveareas.com – helping people to help themselves. This site offers free resources, practitioner workshops on using self-help and other resources to help support practitioners in their use of the approach.

A note about copyright

The materials in this book, once purchased in book form, may be copied by the user as many times as required for use by themselves or (if a practitioner) in clinical practice or in training.

Acknowledgements

No set of materials such as this could have been written by only one person. The creation and further development of this course would not have been possible without the support, feedback and stimulation I have received from a variety of colleagues over the years. I also owe an immense debt to the comments and feedback of people using these materials and to colleagues who have attended various training workshops and asked difficult questions that have helped test and improve the approach.

My colleagues within the Glasgow SPIRIT and START training teams and also the Living Life to the Full trainers have provided invaluable feedback – Theresa O'Brien, Sandra Johnston, Anne Joice, Catriona Kent, Ann McCreath, Willie Munro, Liz Rafferty and Eileen Riddoch. I wish to especially thank Dr Frances Cole who started this all off by commissioning me to write the course in the first place and in coordinating the initial feedback on the content of the workbooks within Calderdale and Kirklees Health Authority.

The Scottish Executive and the Centre for Change and Innovation have helped fund the further development of the Living Life to the Full website and the online practitioners training course at www.fiveareas.com. Both websites have been expertly supported by the programming and design efforts of Ian Mayer at Mirata Ltd (www.mirata.ltd.uk).

The illustrations in the workbooks were produced by Keith Chan (kchan75@hotmail.com); most are copyright of Media Innovations Limited and used with permission. Thanks too to the staff at Hodder Headline, who have supported the development of the series of new five areas materials that are being released over the next few years.

Finally, I wish to thank my wife Alison and my children Hannah and Andrew who have supported me during the writing of this book.

Dr Chris Williams

Part 1
Understanding why I feel as I do

Starting out: using the course materials . . . and how to keep going if you feel stuck

Dr Chris Williams

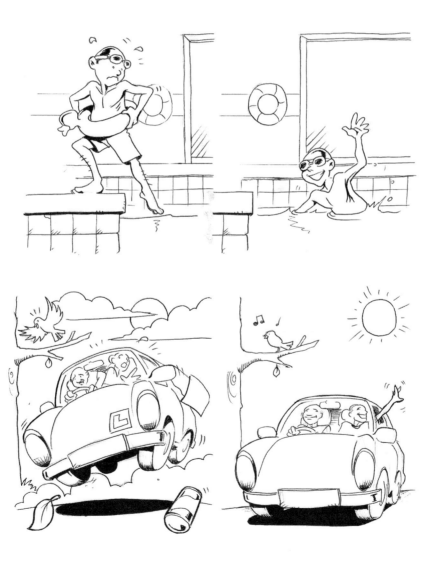

A Five Areas Approach
Helping you to help yourself
www.livinglifetothefull.com

Section 1   Introduction

This workbook covers:

- An introduction to the course.
- A brief introduction to low mood and depression.
- An overview of the **five areas approach** to understanding low mood.
- Optional information on how to overcome common blocks/problems in making changes.
- How to get the most out of the course workbooks.
- A summary and practice plan.
- An appendix with a learning/achievement record sheet.

These workbooks have been written by a practitioner who has many years of experience in using and teaching the cognitive behaviour therapy (CBT) approach. This is one of the most effective ways of improving low mood and depression. It can also be effective for problems such as anxiety, tension and stress that are also commonly present when we feel low. The course will help you to understand more about how your problems are affecting you. The course will also teach you some key skills that you can use to improve how you feel.

So what is cognitive behaviour therapy?

CBT was first developed in the 1950s by an American doctor, Professor Aaron Beck. Beck had become dissatisfied with existing forms of psychological treatment that focused mainly on our early lives. Instead, he wanted to focus on changing how we feel now. He noticed that when we feel down, we tend to see things negatively. We become critical of ourselves and tend to misinterpret everything in a negative way. Beck also noticed that during times of upset we alter what we do and how we relate to others. Some of these changes backfire and worsen how we feel. Based on this work, CBT was developed. CBT is a **self-help form of psychotherapy**. It helps people to make practical changes in their thoughts and actions in order to improve how they feel. It provides people with new tools to make these changes.

The CBT approach is attractive to many people because it is practical and focuses on problems they face now. At the same time, it can help us to understand and change symptoms that have their origins in past experiences. CBT is also one of the most effective ways of improving low mood. In particular, this course aims to provide access to the CBT approach by using an everyday language that is easily understood and put into practice.

The use of CBT self-help approaches has been endorsed by the National Institute for Clinical Excellence (NICE; www.nice.org.uk) as a recommended treatment option for low mood and depression. But why use CBT self-help such as this course?

Why use these workbooks?

In deciding whether this approach is for you, it might help to know that medical treatments for low mood and depression traditionally have fallen into two main approaches – medication and psychological treatments. Both have been shown to be effective. However, clinical guidelines and research now show clearly that antidepressant medication should not be used for symptoms of mild depression; instead, psychological treatments should be tried first. Even for more severe depression, psychological treatments such as CBT are recommended alongside medication. Self-help materials based on CBT principles are increasingly available and are popular with both the general public and healthcare practitioners. Most bookshops have large self-help sections, and self-help books are often among the top ten bestselling books. People like to use self-help for all sorts of reasons. The most common reason is that it provides access to key information and skills. **You, the reader, are in control** – and you can work on things at a time that suits you rather than a healthcare practitioner. Time and time again people surprise themselves by the amount of change they can make themselves using a self-help approach.

The self-help approach can be used along with medication where this is needed. The workbooks may also be used by people who are feeling anxious or experiencing many other common mental health problems. This is because the course teaches skills that can be applied in a whole range of life situations.

Picking the right time for the approach

In general, the following would suggest that it might **not** be helpful to use this sort of approach at this time:

- You just aren't the sort of person who likes to use workbooks or self-help approaches.
- You have severe depression, which causes very poor concentration and low energy levels, making reading and the use of written materials just too difficult at the moment. (But note: they can always be used at a later time.)

The next section will help you to find out more about depression and low mood.

Section 2   A brief introduction to low mood and depression

Feeling fed up and low in mood is a normal part of life. When difficulties or upsetting events occur, it is not unusual to feel down and stop enjoying things. Likewise when good things happen, we may experience happiness, pleasure and a sense of really being able to achieve things in life. The reasons for low mood are usually clear. They include stressful situations, relationship difficulties, feeling let down by someone, financial difficulties, unforeseen events or some other practical problem. Most of the time the drop in mood lasts for only a short period of time, and then we 'bounce back'.

Occasionally, however, this 'depressed' feeling worsens and dominates our life. When someone feels like this for more than two weeks, doctors call it a **depressive illness**. It is important to say that depression is very common and can affect anyone. You will find out more about this in the workbook *Understanding why I feel as I do*.

The following checklist will help you to identify whether you have any of the common symptoms of depression:

 Low mood/depression checklist

Situation, relationship and practical problems:

Have I faced any recent significant life losses or life challenges?	Yes ☐	No ☐	Sometimes ☐
Have problems been building up and now they seem overwhelming?	Yes ☐	No ☐	Sometimes ☐

Altered thinking:

Have I become much more critical of myself?	Yes ☐	No ☐	Sometimes ☐
Am I very negative about things in general?	Yes ☐	No ☐	Sometimes ☐
Am I sometimes hopeless about the future and the possibility of recovery?	Yes ☐	No ☐	Sometimes ☐
Am I finding it more difficult to keep my mind focused on things?	Yes ☐	No ☐	Sometimes ☐

Altered feelings:

Do I feel depressed or weepy?	Yes ☐	No ☐	Sometimes ☐
Is my ability to enjoy things less than normal?	Yes ☐	No ☐	Sometimes ☐

Altered physical symptoms/bodily sensations:

Has there been a change in my appetite, energy levels or sleep?	Yes ☐	No ☐	Sometimes ☐

Altered behaviour:

Have I begun to reduce or stop doing things that previously gave me a sense of pleasure or achievement?	Yes ☐	No ☐	Sometimes ☐

| Have I begun to be less socially active/stay in more? | Yes ☐ | No ☐ | Sometimes ☐ |
| Have I begun to lose confidence in doing things? | Yes ☐ | No ☐ | Sometimes ☐ |

If you have answered yes to questions in most of the five areas listed in bold, you are likely to be experiencing a depressive illness. Depression will be affecting your **thinking**, **feelings**, **body**, **behaviour** and **social activities** to a significant extent. If you have many yes answers, please talk to your healthcare practitioner, if you haven't already done so, to find out more about this. They will be able to help you to work out whether you are experiencing a depressive disorder.

If you have fewer yes answers, you may not be experiencing depression or you could have a milder form of depression.

 Finally, if you wish to measure your levels of anxiety and depression using a free online mood questionnaire, you can register for free on the support site for this course at www.livinglifetothefull.com.

The emotion balance

In times of distress we often feel overwhelmed and struggle to cope. We tend to dwell on difficulties so that the problems build up in our mind. At the same time we usually **underplay** our own ability to deal with the problem. This tendency to dwell on problems also means that we not only feel down but also worry about things. Depression and anxiety therefore often occur together, with most people noticing both problems at the same time. Other words we may use to describe this worry are 'stress', 'tension' and 'fear'. If this is the case for you, then tackling the low mood may result in a marked improvement in your stress levels too.

Let's look at the emotion balance and think about how it may relate to you. Normally, we feel able to cope with the problems we face. In a situation where we feel in balance, we know we can deal with our problems.

In contrast, during times of low mood and distress, this balance is upset. An unhelpful focus on problems and difficulties occurs. Our problems are seen as too large or overwhelming, and we think we cannot cope. In both situations, the emotion balance is upset, and the result is we feel increasing distress.

Out of balance – rising distress

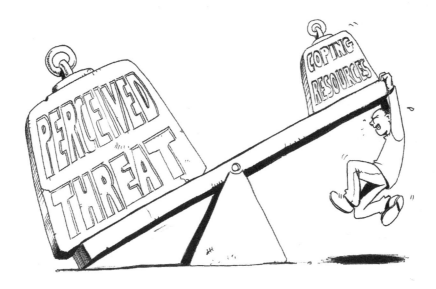

Do I feel in balance at the moment?   Yes ☐ No ☐ Sometimes ☐

The emotion balance has important implications. It means that **it is not the situation or problem alone that causes us to feel down or stressed; instead, it is how we interpret it.** This is not to say that practical problems and difficulties don't need to be dealt with – they do. However, dwelling on problems and getting things out of perspective is not an effective solution.

Let's move on now to find out more about how the five areas approach can help you understand the impact of lowered mood. A first key step is becoming convinced that the approach is worth using. In the next section, you can test whether the approach will be able to help you work out the answer to 'Why do I feel as I do?'

Section 3 Understanding low mood using the five areas assessment approach

One helpful way of understanding the impact that low mood and depression have on us is to consider the ways they can affect different areas of our life. A **five areas assessment** approach can help us to do this by examining in detail the following five important aspects of our lives:

- Life situation, relationships, practical resources and problems.
- Altered thinking.
- Altered feelings (also called moods or emotions).
- Altered physical symptoms/bodily sensations.
- Altered behaviour or activity levels, including both helpful and unhelpful responses that can backfire on how we feel.

Think about how the five areas assessment can help us understand the following two situations involving John and Anne.

 EXAMPLE

John's wallet

John and Anne have been friends for several years. Both now are finding it difficult to cope for different reasons.

John is going shopping. As he gets ready to leave home, he suddenly realises that he cannot find his wallet (= **life situation/practical problem**). He jumps immediately to the very worst conclusion that his wallet and credit cards were stolen the last time he was out. He fears that the thieves will run up a large debt on his credit cards (= **altered thinking**). This makes him feel very anxious and tense. What he thinks has affected how he feels (= **altered feelings/emotions**). He begins to notice a sick feeling in his stomach and a strong sense of tension throughout his body. He feels quite sweaty and clammy and notices a pressure in his head (= **altered physical sensations**). He immediately contacts his credit-card company and bank to cancel the cards (= **altered behaviour**).

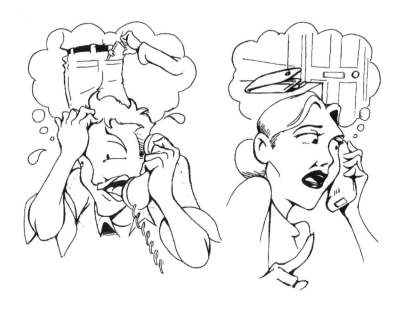

John then phones his friend Anne to tell her what has happened. She is sympathetic and encourages him to try to remember where he last saw the wallet. Anne suggests that he looks around the house to see whether he can find it. John thanks her. He is pleased that he called Anne because he feels a little better as a result. He promises to phone Anne that evening to let her know whether he has found the wallet.

Later that day, he finds the wallet in his coat pocket. He realises he had forgotten he put it there yesterday. He then tries to avoid seeing or talking to Anne, because he is worried that she will think he is a right fool. He doesn't phone her back that evening to let her know he has found the wallet. John feels angry at himself and beats himself up mentally about it ('You idiot!'), leading him to feel really low and down.

John interpreted the situation in both an **extreme** and **unhelpful** way. He ended up feeling both worried and very down in his mood. He is now unable to use his credit cards as a result of his unfounded fears.

The following diagram summarises John's five areas assessment. This helps him look at five areas of experience to help him make sense of what happens when he has a strong emotion. Here is John looking at the changes that occur when he feels really anxious and worried:

John's wallet

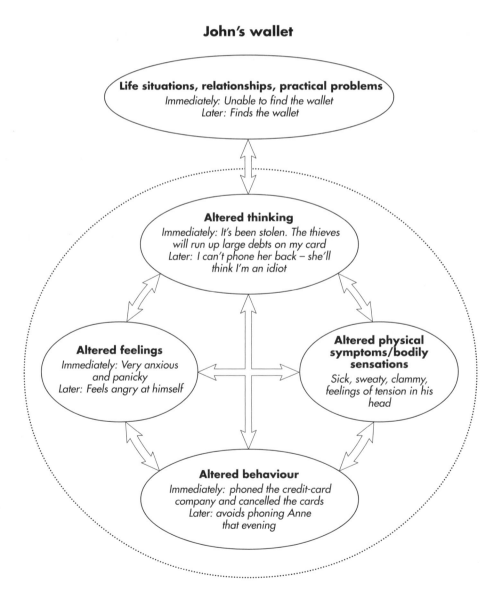

Life situations, relationships, practical problems
Immediately: Unable to find the wallet
Later: Finds the wallet

Altered thinking
Immediately: It's been stolen. The thieves will run up large debts on my card
Later: I can't phone her back – she'll think I'm an idiot

Altered feelings
Immediately: Very anxious and panicky
Later: Feels angry at himself

Altered physical symptoms/bodily sensations
Sick, sweaty, clammy, feelings of tension in his head

Altered behaviour
Immediately: phoned the credit-card company and cancelled the cards
Later: avoids phoning Anne that evening

The five areas diagram shows that what we think about a situation or problem may affect how we feel physically and emotionally and may alter what we do (behaviour or activity levels). Look at the arrows in the diagram. Each of the five areas (situation, relationship or practical problems, thinking, emotional and physical feelings, and behaviour changes) affects the others.

Think about how well John's reactions in the diagram can be explained using this approach. Can times that you have felt worse be explained in this way? The same approach can be used to look at the impact of anxiety and any other strong emotion such as low mood, anger, guilt and shame.

You may find the diagram difficult to understand at first, or you may not be sure whether it applies to you. The next questions will help you to begin to think about how each area affects the others. By looking at John's responses, you can then begin to think about how this might also affect you.

 CHOICE POINT

If you are not sure about how to answer the next questions, skip them and move to the example *Anne fears a broken friendship* below.

(?) How do John's **thoughts, feelings** and **physical reactions** fit together? Look at those three boxes in John's five areas assessment. How does what he **thought** about the situation affect how he **felt** about it?

✎

....

....

....

(?) Look again at the thoughts and behaviour boxes in John's five areas assessment. How do John's **thoughts** and **behaviour** fit together? How does what he **thought** about the situation affect what he **did** about it?

✎

....

....

....

(?) What do you think of John's interpretation of what had happened (immediately **jumping to the very worst conclusion** that the wallet was stolen and his prediction that Anne will think badly of him – sometimes called **mind-reading**)?

✎

....

....

....

? How could John have altered how he felt and what he did (immediately cancelling the cards and then failing to phone Anne after he found the wallet again)?

✎

....

....

....

---

e.g. **EXAMPLE**

Anne fears a broken friendship

John promised to phone Anne to let her know whether he found his wallet. Anne is wondering why he hasn't phoned (= **life situation/relationships**). She begins to worry that she may have sounded irritable towards him. The fact is that he has phoned her before in similar situations when he can't find something important. She knows that he usually finds the lost object after a proper search. 'Oh dear,' she thinks. 'Did I sound a bit irritable towards John?' She worries that she might not have been supportive enough. She blames herself for upsetting him and not being a good friend (= **altered thinking**). She feels guilty and low because of this (= **altered feelings/emotions**). That night Anne can't relax (= **altered physical sensations**), and she lies awake anxiously, worrying that she has upset John and harmed their friendship. She decides not to phone him for a few days (= **altered behaviour**) because she is not sure how he might react if she really has upset him. Perhaps he will break off their friendship?

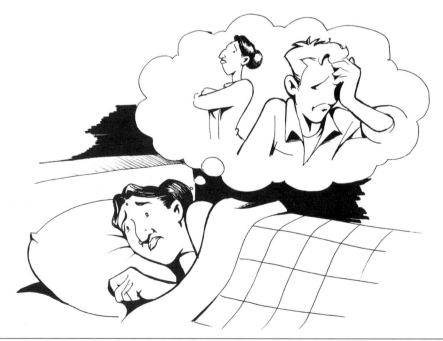

The following diagram summarises Anne's five areas assessment:

Anne's reaction

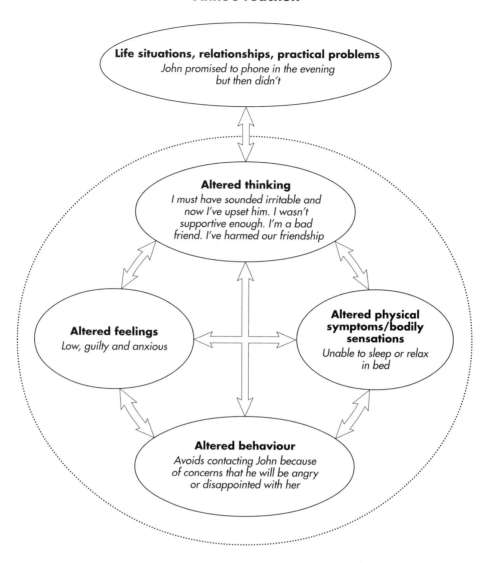

Life situations, relationships, practical problems
John promised to phone in the evening but then didn't

Altered thinking
I must have sounded irritable and now I've upset him. I wasn't supportive enough. I'm a bad friend. I've harmed our friendship

Altered feelings
Low, guilty and anxious

Altered physical symptoms/bodily sensations
Unable to sleep or relax in bed

Altered behaviour
Avoids contacting John because of concerns that he will be angry or disappointed with her

💡 LEARNING POINT

You can go round the diagram repeatedly in many different directions rather than just clockwise. This can build an even larger problem. To understand this more, please answer the following five questions. You can skip them if you find them too hard.

(?) How do Anne's **thoughts, feelings** and **physical reactions** fit together?

✎

....

....

....

(?) How do Anne's **thoughts** and **behaviour** fit together?

✎

....

....

....

(?) Did her fear that she had upset John affect how she **felt** and what
she **did**?   Yes ☐   No ☐

(?) Were her thoughts that she had upset John accurate and helpful?

✎

....

....

....

(?) How could she have checked out what John really thought?

✎

....

....

....

In these two examples, the person's fears (**jumping to the very worst conclusion** and **mind-reading** what the other person thought) led them to feel more anxious and eventually lowered their mood. Something that took only a few minutes on the phone resulted in much unnecessary worry and distress over the following hours because of the conclusions to which they both jumped. It also affected, unhelpfully, how they behaved. In spite of their concerns, neither Anne nor John actually did anything to check out how their friend had really reacted. If they had, they would have realised quite how unhelpful and wrong their fears were.

LEARNING POINT

These examples also show that it is not necessarily the events themselves that cause upset, but the **interpretation** the person makes of the event. When we feel low or anxious about things, we tend to develop more extreme, negative and unhelpful ways of thinking (**unhelpful thinking**). These thoughts can build up out of all proportion and unhelpfully affect how we feel and what we do. This can keep our feelings of upset going.

Look at the table below. This summarises the original way in which John and Anne reacted. It also shows an alternative way in which they could have reacted if they had interpreted what happened differently.

The impact of other ways of seeing things

Situation	Thought	Feeling/physical sensations	Altered behaviour
John's original reaction: 'I can't find the wallet'	'It's been stolen!'	Anxious, panicky, sick, sweaty, clammy; later angry at himself when he finds it	Cancels credit cards; later avoids phoning Anne
John's alternative reaction: same situation – 'I can't find the wallet'	'Oh, John! You'd lose your own head if it wasn't fixed on. I'll probably find it like last time. I just need to have a look for it'	Quite relaxed	Looks around the house and finds his wallet – and also his mobile, which he 'lost' last week
Anne's original reaction: 'John promised to phone this evening, but he didn't'	'I've upset him/been a bad friend'	Low, guilty, anxious, unable to sleep or relax	Avoids John in case he is angry with her
Anne's alternative reaction: same situation – 'John promised to phone this evening, but he didn't'	'He must have found it or he'd have phoned me again. That John! I do love him dearly. I'm just surprised he hasn't lost his mobile yet'	Thinks fondly of John	Phones him the next day to find out that he has indeed found the wallet. They have a laugh and arrange to meet up for a coffee

These examples of Anne and John point to some important changes such as altered thinking and behaviour that may also be present in our own lives. By changing our unhelpful thinking and unhelpfully altered behaviour, we can improve how we feel.

You will have the opportunity in the workbook *Understanding why I feel as I do* to see whether the five areas approach can help you understand how you are feeling.

 IMPORTANT POINT

You may be tempted to move on to that workbook immediately. I'd really like to encourage you to first read the rest of this workbook first though. This covers how to plan to use the workbooks on a regular basis. It will also help you to overcome common problems that can block or undermine your use of the workbooks.

Other changes commonly seen in low mood and depression

You have already seen the range of ways in which Anne and John responded to upsetting circumstances. We now discuss some other common changes seen at times of low mood.

Worry and stress

Worrying thoughts are common in low mood.

In worry, we anxiously go over things again and again in a way that is unhelpful because it does not actually help us sort out the difficulties that we are worried about.

Sometimes the worry may be out of all proportion. For example, something that originally happened in a few moments, such as something someone said to you, can be on your mind for much of the following days or weeks. This can add up to days or even weeks of worry over the following months. You may also find that you are feeling worried without being too sure what you are worrying about.

Panic attacks

Sometimes anxiety can rise to such a high level that we feel so mentally and physically tense and unwell that we stop what we are doing and try to leave or escape the situation. Sometimes we may feel paralysed into inactivity like a rabbit caught in the headlamps of a car and freeze, expecting disaster to strike at any moment. This feeling of acute fear, dread or terror is called a **panic attack**. Panic attacks rarely last for more than 20–30 minutes. This is because physiologically it takes the body time to create, store and release the chemical adrenalin. Although we may continue to feel anxious, that very high level of terror and panic drops off as the body is physically unable to keep releasing adrenalin at the same high rate.

During panic, there are strong beliefs that something terrible or catastrophic is happening right now. Common fears include 'I'm going to faint', 'I'm going to suffocate', 'I'm going to collapse', 'I'm going to have a stroke' and 'I'm going to have a heart attack'. Sometimes the fear is of **going mad** or **losing control**. The fear is always immediately threatening, scary and catastrophic. We may then become overly aware of the anxious fears, quickly stop what we are doing and hurry away from the situation.

Obsessional thoughts

Obsessional thoughts can also occur during times of low mood. These describe a situation where the person repeatedly notices that upsetting thoughts pop into their mind again and again and again, even when they try hard not to think them. A milder form of this experience is quite common. Many people have had the experience of noticing that a tune seems to get 'stuck' and goes round and round in their mind for a time before eventually disappearing. In most cases this is seen as either OK (the person just hums along) or slightly annoying and frustrating. Eventually it stops.

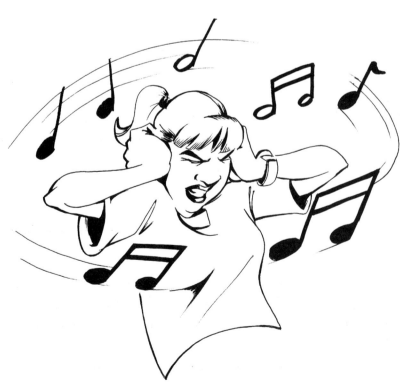

The big difference is that the thought **continues** to go round and round for a very long time in spite of the person making efforts to stop thinking it. Because the thoughts are so distressing, the person becomes overly aware of them and tries hard not to think the upsetting thoughts.

Common obsessional thoughts include a fear of hurting or damaging others in some way or of causing harm through not having done something. The person is worried that something really bad will happen as a result. They may know rationally that no such harm is really likely to occur, and yet the worrying fears dominate their thinking and intrude into their mind. Sometimes obsessive thinking results in the person becoming crippled by doubt about a particular issue, or they feel compelled to repeat certain compulsive actions, for example cleaning or checking things repeatedly.

Getting help for worry, stress, panic, obsessions and compulsions

This course contains many workbooks that will help you tackle anxiety, improve sleep, challenge worrying thoughts and rebuild activity. Free online relaxation resources are available at www.livinglifetothefull.com. You can find out more about panic attacks, obsessions and compulsions in detail in the companion book *Overcoming Anxiety: A Five Areas Approach*.

Next steps

You are most likely to be able to make helpful and positive changes in your life if **you** are in charge of what you read. To get the most from the course, you need to work it through by trying out what you learn in your own life.

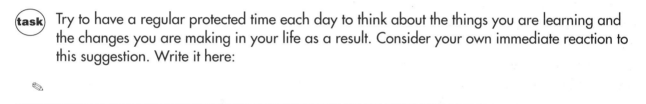 Try to have a regular protected time each day to think about the things you are learning and the changes you are making in your life as a result. Consider your own immediate reaction to this suggestion. Write it here:

....

....

....

Completing the tasks set out in each workbook is an important part of changing. It is the day-to-day practice of these tasks that will help you get better. This will encourage you to bring the workbooks into your everyday week to help you to **stop, think and reflect** on how you are feeling. You may believe at first that nothing is changing, but slowly you will notice positive changes.

CHOICE POINT

You may have had all sorts of reactions. If you feel that making such a commitment will be relatively easy, then feel free to skip the next section, which addresses ways of overcoming low motivation and blocks to progress, and go on to Section 5.

Most of us, however, aren't always so positive. We are even more likely to have doubts when we feel low. If we think negatively 'The course won't work for me', or 'It's going to be too hard', or 'I won't understand the workbooks', then this may stop you using this approach. In this case, keep reading Section 4, which follows.

Section 4   Overcoming blocks to progress

An important thing to bear in mind is that motivation is low during times of distress. When people feel low or anxious it can be very difficult to make changes. You may be sleeping poorly, have low energy levels, be in pain or tired, find it difficult focusing your mind, and struggle to be motivated to change. However, this can be overcome by using several strategies to build your motivation to change.

Building your motivation to change

 EXPERIMENT

Take some time to write yourself one of the following letters. Try to do this now before moving on, even if it seems difficult.

- **If you aren't really sure that you are ready for change**, imagine it is ten years in the future. Things have gone on unchanged, exactly as they are now. Write yourself a letter giving yourself advice and encouragement about why you need to make changes now.

- **If you have already decided that you want change but need some encouragement**, you may prefer to write the following letter: imagine it is ten years in the future. You have made important changes in your life and recovered fully. Things are much better and you have achieved many of the goals you set yourself. Write yourself an encouraging letter about why you need to make changes now.

....

....

....

....

....

....

....

....

....

....

....

....

....

....

....

Learning to swim

Sometimes we forget how difficult it is to learn new information or skills that you now take for granted. Think about some of the skills you have learned over the years. For example, if you can drive or swim, think back to your first driving or swimming lesson. It is unlikely you were very good at it that first time, and yet with practice you developed the knowledge and skills needed to drive or swim. It may have been difficult at the time, but you managed it. You can overcome low mood and tension in the same way. It may seem difficult at first, but keep practising what you learn.

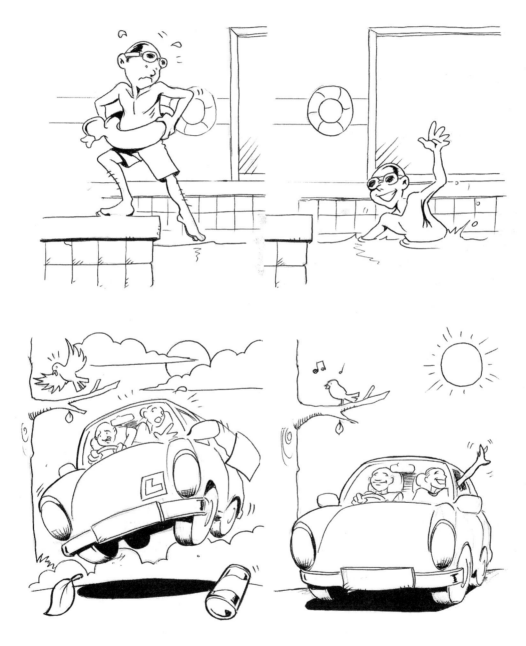

(task) Write down some other things you have learned that took time:

....

....

....

IMPORTANT POINT

You can't expect to be able to swim immediately. You may need to start at the shallow end and practise first. Use these workbooks in a similar way. Pace what you do and don't jump immediately and enthusiastically into the deep end.

Having realistic expectations

It's important not to approach this course either too positively or too negatively. It would be untrue to claim that if you use this course, you can guarantee results. What can be guaranteed is that the CBT approach has helped many thousands of people, and the workbooks teach clinically proven approaches. One aim of the course is that you will feel better in many important ways, but the course also aims to help you to learn some interesting and helpful things along the way.

Tackling the things that might block you from using the course

A number of issues often seem to cause problems in planning to use the workbooks. Some of the most common are:

'I've no time'

It may be that you think that you have so many external pressures, such as relationships and the demands of others, that you can't look after your own needs. Getting better should be a priority. It is important both for you and for those around you that you spend time to allow yourself to get better.

Imagine you had a close friend who was feeling down and distressed. They didn't like how they felt, and you knew that it was affecting them in lots of different ways. What advice would you give them if they said 'I don't have time'?

If we would give them sensible advice to make some time, could we take that same advice ourselves?

'I feel too down to do this now'

Sometimes in severe depression, it might not be the right time to use this sort of workbook. You can always plan to come back to the workbooks at a later stage if you are finding things too much. A practical point here is that your concentration can limit the amount of time you can spend at present. If you find you can't concentrate for long, then just try to read a single page or paragraph and go at a pace you can manage. You should also discuss the treatment options available with your doctor.

'I'll never change'

One of the biggest blocks to getting better is not believing that you can change. If you believe that change is not possible and decide to do nothing as a result, then you may end up missing out on real benefits. Change is possible. Most people find that this initial negative response proves incorrect and they gain much more from the course than they initially expect. Could this be true for you?

Again, imagine your friend has told you they believed they would never change from a time of low mood. They need encouragement, particularly when they believe nothing can change.

(?) What would you say to them? Write it down here:

✎

....

....

....

If you would offer helpful and positive advice to a friend, then why not also offer it to yourself?

Other blocking thoughts

Try to think about whether you are being negative or critical of specific aspects of the workbooks. The following comments by past users of the course may help you:

Blocking thought	Reply
'They are too long'	Try to break down things so you read it one section or even one page at a time. You can physically do that by tearing out pages and aiming to read them if this helps
'I don't like reading'	Other versions of the course are available, including an audio version, an online version at www.livinglifetothefull.com and a further education college course version
'I don't like the cartoons'	The cartoons make up only some of the book. We have tried to use cartoons that build upon the text. We welcome feedback, but if for now you don't find them helpful ignore them – or even cross them out – and instead try to focus on the text
'I don't want to answer questions'	Answers don't have to be long. It may seem strange at first, but the more practice you have doing this the easier it will become. Why not give it a go?
'I don't like the book: it's just not my way of working'	We are all different. Not everyone likes the same books. If you've given it a good go, then maybe this style of book isn't one for you. Other recommended books that are longer or shorter and use different writing styles are available at www.livinglifetothefull.com

Relabel what you are doing

Sometimes people talk themselves out of using the course. You may find reading or using the workbooks too hard or unattractive in some other way. You may find it helpful to think about the course in a different way, for example as **reading** or **self-discovery** of **new life skills**. Other people may prefer to view the course as a **prescription** to be taken each day. Or, if you're the sort of person who likes to exercise (I don't!), try thinking of it as some sort of **life workout** or **physiotherapy for the mind**.

But I still don't feel like it!

Sometimes it can be really hard to get going with making the changes needed to improve how we feel. You've made it this far – which is great. **Choose change**, even if you don't feel like it. Try to do something small first. Put your toes in the water.

EXPERIMENT

Even if you have doubts about the course or your ability to use it effectively, try to give it a go. This will help you to test it out in practice in your own life. If you still find the course doesn't help after you've given it a good go, then that would be a sensible time to try something different.

You might find it useful to come back from time to time to work through this section if you find your motivation to continue the course varies.

 As a final task for this section, try to keep a record of your successes and things that you are learning as you go through the course. Write these down on the *Record sheet: things I am learning and achieving* at the end of this workbook. This record will help you build your motivation for change.

Section 5 How to get the most out of the workbooks

Well done! You've got to the last section – and you're still reading. That's a very important achievement. So many people who want to change find it difficult starting out. Here are some suggestions on building on this first step during the rest of the course.

Planning how and when to use the workbooks

Take time to read the workbooks at your own pace. It can be very helpful to set aside a clear time each day to go through the workbooks. Doing this on a regular basis – even if it is just a short time to begin with – is important. It is often helpful to actively plan this into your day and diary rather than just trying to fit it in at some point.

You may find the following planning task helpful in making this regular commitment. Use it to help you plan how to use the next workbook. This workbook will then help you decide which other workbooks you might need to use.

When am I going to plan to read the workbook *Understanding why I feel as I do*? Is reading some of it every day practical for you? If not, then is every other day more realistic? Many people with low mood notice they feel at their worst first thing in the morning. Using the workbooks after lunch or in the late afternoon or early evening may be the best time for you.

....

....

....

How much will I read? Many people find it helpful to aim to read just one section at a time. Make sure that you stop, think and reflect by answering the questions as you do this.

....

....

....

Is this **realistic, practical** and **achievable**? You know your own life and its various demands and commitments.

....

....

....

(?) What **problems** and **difficulties** could block or prevent me doing this, and how can I overcome these?

✎

....

....

....

Getting into the mood

Doing something physical can help you get started.

We often notice reduced activity when we feel low. You may be doing very little during the day and find it hard to see yourself making any changes. A good start to using the workbooks is to do something physical first. For example, get up, and walk around the room or up and down the stairs. Then sit down on a different chair: try an upright kitchen chair that forces you to sit up rather than slump back. Then start reading the workbook.

Using the workbooks

Each workbook focuses on a different type of problem commonly experienced during times of upset. You don't have to start at the beginning of the course and read it through page by page. Instead, you can choose those areas of your life that you want to work on changing. Each workbook can be read alone or in addition to the other workbooks in the course. A key principle is that the workbooks are about change. They are **work** books and require some work and effort.

To help you make this change:

- Have a pen on hand as you read. Try to **answer all the questions** asked. The process of having to **stop, think and reflect** upon how the questions might be relevant to you is crucial to you getting better.

- **Write down** your own notes in the margins or in the *My notes* area at the end of the workbook to help you remember useful information. Some people like to keep to hand a diary or the *Record sheet: things I am learning and achieving* (page 28) to help them remember key things they are learning. **Review your notes** regularly so that you apply what you have learned.

- Once you have read through the entire workbook once, put it to one side and then **reread it** a few days later. It may be that different parts of the workbook become clearer or seem more useful on the second reading.

- Use the workbooks to **build upon the help** you receive in other ways, such as other helpful reading, talking to friends, self-help organisations, a practitioner and support groups.

- **Respond with actions** that build upon your reading. Try out what you read in the workbooks from the word go. If you learn anything new, then try it out and see whether it helps. A specific section at the end of each workbook will help you to decide how to do this. Have you any ideas so far?

- Jot down any questions or things you are unsure of as you go along. This will help you remember. You can then come back to them later on, or discuss them with a friend, relative, self-help group or practitioner.

Finding extra support

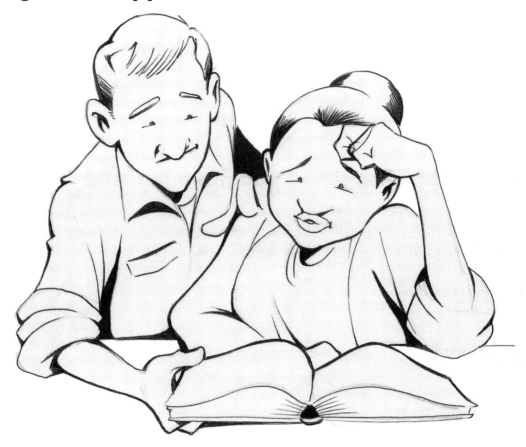

Everyone is different. Some people prefer to use the workbooks alone. Others prefer to discuss what they are learning with another person, such as a practitioner, a trusted family member or a friend. This can be helpful because:

- It can help keep us on track.
- Someone else is there to encourage us if we are struggling.
- It can be useful to talk through some of the issues as you go through the workbooks.

Think about whether there is someone you know and trust who can offer helpful advice. You might go through your answers to the workbooks together, or you might keep your answers private and discuss only some of the course content. The workbook *Information for families and friends: how can I offer support?* has been written specifically to help others help you.

 The online course at www.livinglifetothefull.com is designed to support readers of this book. The online teaching sessions include all the main elements of this book plus additional handouts and resources such as relaxation tapes and online discussion forums to swap ideas and find encouragement from others. The further development of the site was sponsored by the Scottish Executive Health Department and the Centre for Change and Innovation in collaboration with Depression Alliance Scotland and is free to everyone, regardless of where they live.

Other sources of support

A large number of supports are available for people facing low mood and depression. These are listed on the website www.livinglifetothefull.com.

Workbook summary

In this workbook, you have covered:
- An introduction to the course.
- A brief introduction to low mood and depression.
- An overview of the **five areas approach** to understanding low mood.
- Optional information on how to overcome common blocks and problems in making changes.
- How to get the most out of the course workbooks.

Putting into practice what you have learned

Experience has shown that you are likely to make more progress if you are able to put into practice what you have learned in the workbook. Each workbook will encourage you to do this by suggesting certain tasks for you to carry out in the following days.

 Copy or tear out the *Record sheet: things I am learning and achieving* at the end of this workbook. At the end of each day, write down at least one thing you have learned or achieved. Spend some time reflecting on this to encourage you as you think about what you've learned. Keep the sheet in a place where you can see it every day and add to it as you go through the workbooks.

Next workbook

It is suggested that you read the workbook *Understanding why I feel as I do* next. This will help you work out which other course workbooks are relevant to you.

A request for feedback

An important factor in the development of the five areas assessment workbooks is that the content is updated on a regular basis based upon feedback from users and practitioners. If there are areas within it that you find hard to understand or seem poorly written, please let us know and we will try to improve things in future. Unfortunately, we are unable to provide any specific replies or advice on treatment. To provide feedback, please contact us by:
- *Website:* www.livinglifetothefull.com.
- *Email:* feedback@livinglifetothefull.com.
- *Post:* Dr Chris Williams, Psychological Medicine, Gartnavel Royal Hospital, 1055 Great Western Road, Glasgow G12 0XH.

Acknowledgements

I wish to thank all those who have commented upon this workbook, especially Marie Chellingsworth, Dr Nicky Dummett, Ann McCreath, Liz Rafferty and Dr Steve Williams.

The cartoon illustrations in the workbooks were produced by Keith Chan, email kchan75@hotmail.com.

My notes

....

....

....

....

....

....

....

....

....

....

....

....

....

....

....

....

....

....

....

....

....

....

....

....

....

....

My notes

....

....

Record sheet: things I am learning and achieving (please copy or tear out)

....

....

....

....

....

....

....

....

....

....

....

....

....

....

....

....

....

....

....

....

....

....

....

....

....

....

Understanding why I feel as I do

Dr Chris Williams

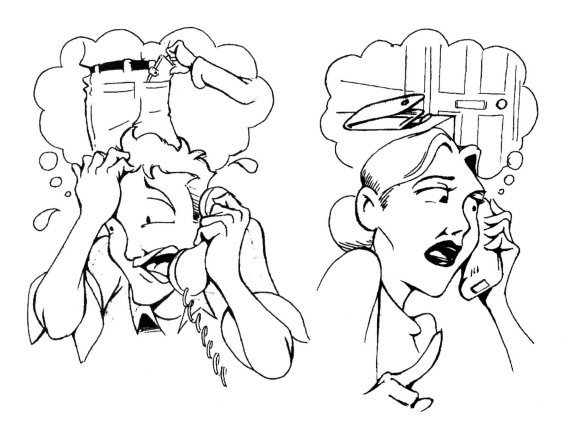

A Five Areas Approach
Helping you to help yourself
www.livinglifetothefull.com

Section *1*   Introduction

The *Overcoming Depression and Low Mood* course is a series of workbooks that will help you to find out about the causes of low mood and to change problem areas of your life so that you begin to feel better.

Before you start:

Think about how much you know about the causes and treatment of low mood. Answer the following questions:

(?) How good is my knowledge about the causes of depression? Make a cross on the line below to record how much you know about the causes of depression:

No knowledge	Excellent knowledge
0	10

(?) How well do I deal with upsetting thoughts or feelings?

Poorly	Very well
0	10

(?) How assertive am I?

Not at all	Very
0	10

(?) How well do I solve practical problems?

Poorly	Very well
0	10

Each of these areas is a **target area for change** in the workbooks. Each workbook focuses on a different area to guide you in making changes that will help you to feel better.

This workbook will cover:

- An introduction to low mood, giving you a chance to consider how your problems have developed.
- How to complete your own five areas assessment, covering your life situation, thoughts, feelings and physical symptoms, and altered behaviour.
- Using your own five areas assessment to help you choose which other course workbooks to use.

The workbooks are designed to help you understand how you feel and to help you plan a step-by-step approach to recovery.

Before you move on to creating your own summary of how low mood is affecting you now, let's spend some time looking at how the problems have developed and where you are now.

How my symptoms have developed

One way of considering how your symptoms have developed is to use a **timeline**. This helps us think about how things have progressed. An example is shown below.

 EXAMPLE

Paul's timeline

Beginning, January: I was working as usual in the factory.

February: Increasing demands at work.

April: Struggling to cope, can't sleep, lying awake worrying about things.

Next 4 months: tried on several medications for depression by my GP.

August: Sick leave from work.

My GP suggests referral to a mental health practitioner.

Told by them I have a depressive disorder.

Today: **Using the course workbooks – I want to make some changes**.

 Use the space on the next page to write in **your own** timeline of the progress of your current problem. Do this to create a general overview of key changes that have happened since your symptoms first started.

Beginning (a time when I last was well)

....

....

....

....

....

....

....

....

....

....

....

....

....

....

....

....

....

....

....

....

Today

By doing this, you can see how things have developed. The good news is that the timeline doesn't stop there. It is possible to improve things. The workbooks in this course can help you to make changes to do this.

CHOICE POINT

If you have recently read the workbook *Starting out: using the course materials . . . and how to keep going if you feel stuck,* you may wish to skip the rest of this section and move to Section 2. Otherwise please read the rest of this section.

How to use the workbooks

This self-assessment workbook normally should be read **over one to two weeks**. It is important to realise this, because this workbook is the longest in the course. Don't pressurise yourself to get through it quickly. It is designed as a workbook – to be worked through slowly. We recommend that any other workbooks are completed every week or so. You can choose to use as many or as few of them as you wish, so that you work to make changes only in areas of your life that are relevant to you. Please also use the workbooks at a pace that is right for you.

The following suggestions will help you get the most out of the course:

- There is a lot of information in each workbook, so the workbooks are divided into clear sections covering each topic. You might find it helpful to read them one section at a time. Keep a pen or pencil with the workbook: you will need it, as there are lots of questions to answer and suggested tasks to do.
- Maybe plan some time during the week that you are going to dedicate to going through the workbooks. If you have lots of other demands in your life, it is important to set aside some time for you and your journey to recovery.
- Try to answer all the questions asked. The process of having to stop, think and reflect on how the questions might be relevant to you is a crucial part of getting better.
- You will probably find that some aspects of each workbook are more useful to you at the moment than others. Write down your own notes of key points in the margins or in the *My notes* area at the back of the workbook to help you remember information that has been helpful. Plan to review your notes regularly to help you apply what you have learned.
- If you are using the workbooks with a healthcare practitioner, jot down any questions you think of as you go along so that you can ask them when you next meet.
- Once you have read through an entire workbook once, you may find it useful to put it on one side and then reread it again a few days later. It may be that different parts of the workbook become clearer or seem more useful on second reading.
- Within each workbook, important areas are labelled as key points. Certain areas that are covered may not be relevant for everyone. Such areas will be identified clearly so that you can choose to skip this optional material if you wish.
- You may wish to discuss the workbooks with a trusted friend or relative. Sometimes the comments of others can help you work out exactly how low mood is affecting you so that you can work together on overcoming the problems. The workbook *Information for families and friends: how can I offer support?* is written for them and can be read at any time while you are doing the course.

What is low mood and depression?

Low mood and feeling fed up, down, blue or depressed are among the many terms used to describe a situation that is a widespread problem for many people. These reactions can feel very difficult to deal with. It can seem as though we are the only people who feel like this. It can be helpful to discover that we are not alone. In fact, low mood and depression can affect **anyone**. At least one in two people develops a depressive disorder at least once in their life. If you, the reader, were the only person feeling like this, then very few books would be published on depression. In fact, books addressing low mood, anxiety and stress are prominently on display in many bookshops.

Low mood and depression are a lot more common than you may think. In the course of each year, around one in ten people experiences high levels of depression. Think back to your class at school. From an average class of 30 students, this means that typically three of your classmates will have problems of low mood this year.

Some well-known people have experienced problems of depression. You may have seen television programmes or read books about their experiences.

When low mood occurs at a high level, it affects the person's mood and thinking, creates a range of physical symptoms in their body, and often causes the person to alter what they do.

When times are difficult . . .

Low mood can make life seem like a real struggle. This is why choosing to commit yourself to the five areas approach is important, and why we recommend using the workbooks together with someone else who can encourage and support you. Taking small steps can make a really big difference to how you feel.

 IMPORTANT POINT

Adjusting just a few small things in your life can result in big benefits. You will find out about some small things you can change as you read this workbook. Try to experiment with these to see what impact they may have on you.

Section 2 **Your own five areas assessment**

In the workbook *Starting out: using the course materials . . . and how to keep going if you feel stuck*, you read a brief introduction to the five areas approach. In this next section, you have an opportunity to complete your own five areas summary of how you feel.

How low mood is affecting you now: your own five areas assessment

Low mood can affect us in many ways. A **five areas assessment** provides a clear summary of the difficulties faced in each of the following areas:

- Life situations, relationships and practical problems.
- Altered thinking, where we are prone to dwell on things and tend to see everything in extreme and unhelpful ways.
- Altered feelings (also called moods or emotions).
- Altered physical symptoms and bodily sensations.
- Altered behaviour or activity levels, with reduced activity, avoidance, and helpful and unhelpful reactions to things.

You have already had the chance to read about Paul and Anne's experience, when Paul thought he had lost his wallet. If you have not read this yet, you may find it helpful to quickly read that example now (see Section 3, page 9 of the workbook *Starting out: using the course materials . . . and how to keep going if you feel stuck*). What follows is an example of how the five areas approach can help us to understand our reactions to things that happen to us.

A five areas assessment can help you begin to understand the links between each of these areas in your own life.

 EXAMPLE

How the five key areas affect each other

Imagine you have had a bad day and are feeling fed up. You decide to go shopping. As you are walking down a road, someone you know walks by and doesn't say anything to you. A number of explanations could be made about what has happened. If you jumped to a very negative conclusion, for example 'They don't like me' (= altered thinking), this might lead to altered emotions (feeling down) and altered behaviour (going home and avoiding other people's company). In the longer term, you might avoid the person or act differently towards them. You might notice some altered physical sensations at the time you felt worse, such as a lack of energy, restlessness or a sinking feeling. Afterwards you may be unable to sleep because of worrying about what happened.

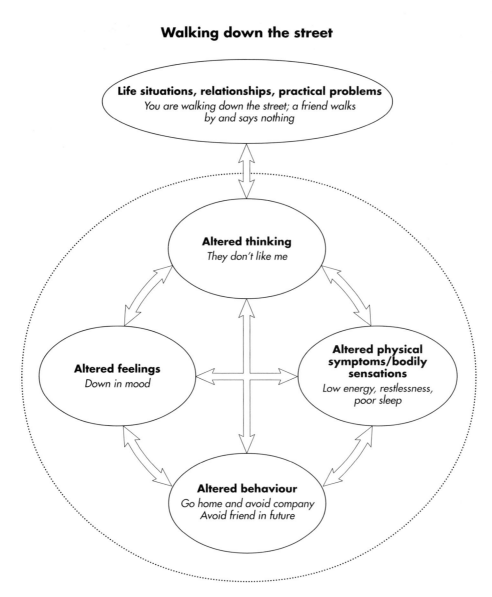

Walking down the street

Life situations, relationships, practical problems
*You are walking down the street; a friend walks
by and says nothing*

Altered thinking
They don't like me

Altered feelings
Down in mood

**Altered physical
symptoms/bodily
sensations**
*Low energy, restlessness,
poor sleep*

Altered behaviour
*Go home and avoid company
Avoid friend in future*

This figure shows that what a person thinks about a situation or problem may affect how they feel physically and emotionally and alter what they do (behaviour or activity). Each of the five areas affects the others.

Explanation

In this instance, what you think might affect how you feel emotionally and physically and what you do. Yet, there may be numerous other explanations as to why your friend may not have said hello. If you had additional information, for example that they were experiencing problems at home, you might have interpreted their walking by differently. If instead your interpretation was 'Maybe they were distracted or upset and just didn't see me' (= **altered thinking**) and you believed this 100 per cent, it's likely that you might feel very differently about what happened. You might be more likely to feel sorry (= **altered feelings**) for the person. You probably wouldn't experience as many or as strong physical symptoms (= **altered physical sensations**), and it is also unlikely that you would avoid seeing them again (= **altered behaviour**). In fact, it's possible you might go out of your way to contact them and ask how they are.

In this example, what you think affects how you feel and what you do. These same reactions are summarised in the table on the next page.

Situation	How we interpret this (thinking)	Altered feelings and behaviour
Original reaction: 'Someone I know walks by and doesn't say anything'	'They don't like me'	Feel down, go home and avoid company
Alternative reaction: Same situation – 'Someone I know walks by and doesn't say anything'	'They have problems at home and were distracted and upset'	Feel sorry for them, perhaps go out of your way to contact them and ask how they are

 KEY POINT

This example also shows that it is not events themselves that cause low mood, but the interpretation that people make of the event. In low mood and depression, the person has more extreme, negative and unhelpful patterns of thinking. These thoughts build up out of all proportion and affect how the person feels and what they do.

 How helpful is this model in understanding how you feel?

Not at all   Extremely helpful

0   10

You now have a chance to look at how depression is affecting you in each of these five areas by carrying out your own five areas assessment. This will help you to find out more about how the five areas approach can help you understand why you feel as you do.

 As you go through the following questions, try hard to stop, think and reflect on your answers. Don't rush though them. Instead, try to answer all the questions so that you are really thinking about how what you read might apply to you.

Area 1: life review – situation, relationship and practical problems contributing to how I feel

All of us from time to time face practical problems and difficulties. The actions of important people around us can also create upsets and difficulties. Practical problems such as relationship or financial difficulties may also be present. When someone faces a large number of problems, they may begin to feel overwhelmed, low and stressed. Dwelling on the problems may worsen things still further and quickly be blown out of all proportion. The person unhelpfully focuses on the problem and mulls it over again and again in a way that doesn't help resolve the problem.

Practical and relationship problems may include:

- Debts, housing or other difficulties.
- Problems in relationships with family, friends, colleagues, etc.
- Other difficult life situations that you face.

Part of your assessment is to consider how these different factors may be affecting you.

Low mood is often linked to **stresses** at home or work (or lack of work, for example unemployment). People who have experienced a relationship split or who have no one to talk to about how they feel are also prone to depression. Young mothers and mothers facing the demands of bringing up many young children are also at greater risk of depression. Other people around us such as relatives and friends can sometimes really help. For example, they may offer practical and helpful support.

Low mood and tension can affect any kind of relationship. We may become confused as to our feelings towards others. We may know intellectually that we love and are loved but feel nothing if we are very depressed. Relationships can lose their interest. Love can feel subdued. For example, a mother may look at her baby and feel nothing – a common symptom in postnatal depression. Similarly, a person with a spiritual faith may find that God seems very distant and struggle to feel His presence when praying.

Situation, relationship and practical problems

 The following checklist summarises several common factors that may be associated with low mood and depression. Are any of these relevant to you?

I have relationship difficulties, such as arguments	Yes ☐	No ☐	Sometimes ☐
My partner doesn't really talk to me or offer me any support	Yes ☐	No ☐	Sometimes ☐
There is no one around who I can really talk to	Yes ☐	No ☐	Sometimes ☐
My children won't do what I tell them	Yes ☐	No ☐	Sometimes ☐
I have difficulties with money worries or debts	Yes ☐	No ☐	Sometimes ☐
There are problems where I live	Yes ☐	No ☐	Sometimes ☐
I am having problems with my neighbours	Yes ☐	No ☐	Sometimes ☐
I don't have a job	Yes ☐	No ☐	Sometimes ☐
I don't enjoy my job	Yes ☐	No ☐	Sometimes ☐
I have difficulties with colleagues at work	Yes ☐	No ☐	Sometimes ☐

Write in any other difficult situations, relationships or practical problems here:

....

....

....

Practical resources and supports

At times of distress, it can sometimes seem that we are aware only of problems and difficulties. We may tend to overlook or downplay our personal strengths. This can lead us to fail to use the possible supports we have around us. There may be a range of supports and resources available to us, including family and trusted friends, having a paid or unpaid role doing something we value, living somewhere we like, or having access to supportive health workers who we find we can work with. Even if at the moment you have few or none of these, there may be other resources that you do have around you. There may be other resources that you have used in the past that have previously proved to be useful aids to feeling better.

Write in any practical resources and supports here:

✎

....

....

....

Summary for area 1: situation, relationship and practical problems

Having answered the questions above:

(?) Overall, do I have problems in this area? Yes ☐ No ☐ Sometimes ☐

(?) Overall, do I have some practical resources in this area? Yes ☐ No ☐ Sometimes ☐

What next?

If this is an area you wish to work on, three of the workbooks in the course will help you to rebalance relationships (*Being assertive* and *Building relationships*) and begin to tackle practical problems (*Practical problem-solving*).

Area 2: altered thinking in low mood and depression

During times of low mood, how we think tends to change. We tend to lose confidence and find it more difficult to make decisions. We may dwell and obsess on things we have done – and things we haven't done. We begin to see everything in extreme and unhelpful ways.

In times of depression, it can seem that everything is viewed in a negative way.

🔑 KEY POINT

You may well notice that you have consistent **unhelpful thinking styles**. Beginning to notice and challenge these is an important part of change on your journey to recovery. These unhelpful thinking styles tend to be:

● Extreme.
● Unhelpful, with a focus on negative things and events, which can worsen how you feel.

🧪 EXPERIMENT

Think about whether you notice these thinking styles in your own life. Read through the table below and tick the column if you have found yourself having thoughts like these in the past two weeks.

Unhelpful thinking style	Some typical ways of seeing things	Tick if you have noticed this thinking style, even if just sometimes
Bias against myself	I'm very self-critical; I overlook my strengths; I see myself as not coping; I don't recognise my achievements	
	The person is very negative and is full of self-blame and critical self-talk. Nothing they do is right. They are their own worst critic, e.g. 'I'm a bad mother', 'I'm useless', 'I mess up everything'	
Putting a negative slant on things (negative mental filter)	I see things through dark-tinted glasses; I see the glass as being half empty rather than half full; whatever I've done in the week it's never enough to give me a sense of achievement; I tend to focus on the bad side of everyday situations	
	Overlooking or downplaying the positive and focusing instead only on the negative side of every situation, e.g. 'The past week was completely awful', 'Nothing went right'	
Having a gloomy view of the future	I think that things will stay bad or get even worse; I tend to predict that things will go wrong; I'm always looking for the next thing to fail	
	Making negative predictions about the future. This may include a loss of hope or having suicidal ideas, e.g. 'He'll leave me if I don't stop being moody and irritable', 'I'm not going to visit my friends – I won't enjoy it'	
Jumping to the worst conclusions	I tend to predict that the very worst outcome will happen; I often think that I will fail terribly badly	
	Sometimes, this process of predicting that the very worst will happen is called **catastrophic thinking**. This can worsen how you feel and unhelpfully alter what you do, e.g. 'If I go into the shop I'll collapse and die'	
Having a negative view about how others see me	I mind-read what others think of me; I often think that others don't like me or think badly of me without evidence	
	Second-guessing or **mind-reading** that others don't like you or see you as weak, boring, stupid or useless. Usually, the person does not actually try to find out whether their fears are true, e.g. 'She thinks I'm not coping'	

Unhelpful thinking style	Some typical ways of seeing things	Tick if you have noticed this thinking style, even if just sometimes
Unfairly taking responsibility for things	I think I should take the blame if things go wrong; I feel guilty about things that are not really my fault; I think I'm responsible for everyone else	
	The person feels pressure for things to go well and blames themselves if things don't go as expected, even if they are not really to blame, e.g. 'I'll ruin the evening for everybody and it will be all my fault', 'It's my fault if my baby doesn't sleep through the night'	
Making extreme statements/rules	I use the words 'always' and 'never' a lot to summarise things; if one bad thing happens to me I often say 'Just typical' because it seems this always happens; I make myself a lot of 'must', 'should', 'ought' or 'got to' rules; I believe I should push myself to do things really well	
	The person makes very strong statements, e.g. 'It was completely useless', even when what actually happened wasn't anywhere near that bad. The person may set themselves impossible targets that no one could possibly meet, e.g. 'I should be able to cope all the time'. This thinking style causes the person to use the words 'should', 'got to', 'must' and 'ought' a lot, as well as 'typical', e.g. 'Just typical: everything always goes wrong'	

 Overall, am I showing at least some extreme and unhelpful thinking?   Yes ☐   No ☐   Sometimes ☐

You might ask why these sorts of thinking matter. They matter because they can:
- Worsen how you feel.
- Alter how you react in ways that worsen things.

Look at the following examples to see some of these links:

Situation	Thoughts that pop into mind	Altered emotional and physical feelings	Altered behaviour
1 You are talking to someone over lunch and the person you talk to looks vacant for a moment	'They find me boring'	Feel low and anxious, physically feel tensed up	May avoid eye contact, answer questions with short replies, try to break off the conversation and leave the table, avoid the person in future
2 You have to do an important task but the machine has jammed	'That always happens: things never go right for me'	Feel frustrated and annoyed, physically feel agitated and restless	Hit the machine hard with your foot – and hurt your toe
3 You are packing your bags at the supermarket checkout and you hear the person behind you tut	'They think I'm not packing things fast enough'	Feel embarrassment and shame, feel very anxious, go red, start sweating and feel a little shaky	Speed up packing the bags and end up fumbling things and dropping one of the bags, which spills everywhere

These situations illustrate different points:
- Each situation can be interpreted in a number of different ways. For example, in situation 1, when the person you talk to looks vacant, it might be that they feel unwell. Or maybe they are feeling anxious and are plucking up courage to ask you something important.
- Everyone reacts differently. For example, in situation 3, if you reacted differently with the thought 'How dare they tut?', you may deliberately slow down your packing. Of course, it's far more likely that the tut wasn't a tut at all – and if it was, it was directed at something completely different.

🔑 KEY POINT

Thinking about things in unhelpful ways once in a while is quite normal and usually doesn't matter so much. We simply feel worse for a time and then move on. However, this ability to put things in perspective and move on tends to be lost during times of low mood. Not only do such thoughts pop into the mind more frequently, but also we become prone to mulling things over. It becomes harder to challenge and put the upsetting thoughts out of mind. We think too much about things we have done or said – or things we haven't done or said. When the focus of our mind is constantly on negative and worrying things, then we tend to feel even worse. We also tend to react in ways that backfire. You will find out more about these unhelpful responses in the next section of this workbook.

What is so unhelpful about these unhelpful thinking styles

All of these ways of thinking can have an **unhelpful** impact on how you feel and what you do:
- **Dwelling on negative or anxious thoughts can be upsetting.** If you are always thinking other people don't like you or think you're no good, or believe the future is really bleak, you are likely to quickly become disheartened, depressed or anxious.
  Negative thinking → lowered or anxious mood.
- **Dwelling on negative or anxious thoughts can worsen how you feel physically.** Low mood can cause physical feelings of low energy, sickness and pain. Sometimes it can also cause a

worsening of existing physical problems, such as migraines, chest pains and tummy aches. Anxious thoughts and mental tension can result in physical tension and other physical symptoms, such as feeling hot, tense, shaky and sweaty.

Negative thinking → physical symptoms.

- **Dwelling on negative or anxious thoughts can unhelpfully alter how you respond.** You may reduce or stop doing things that previously gave you a sense of pleasure or achievement, or you may start doing things that actually worsen how you feel. For example, sometimes people experiencing low mood may stop visiting friends and start drinking too much alcohol in an attempt to block out how they feel.

  Negative thinking → patterns of unhelpful behaviour.

Summary for area 2: altered thinking in low mood and depression

Having answered the questions above:

(?) Overall, do I have problems in this area?   Yes ☐   No ☐   Sometimes ☐

What next?

If this is an area you wish to work on, the workbook *Noticing and changing extreme and unhelpful thinking* can help you to identify and change these ways of thinking.

Area 3: altered feelings/mood in low mood and depression

In low mood and depression, a person may notice changes in how they feel with:

- Low mood and a profound lack of enjoyment or pleasure in things.
- Guilt, worry, stress, tension, anxiety or panic.
- Anger or irritability with yourself or others.
- Shame or embarrassment with yourself or with what you have done.

(?) What emotional changes have you noticed over the past two weeks?

Low or sad	Yes ☐	No ☐	Sometimes ☐
Reduced/no sense of pleasure in things	Yes ☐	No ☐	Sometimes ☐
Loss of all feelings/noticing no feelings at all	Yes ☐	No ☐	Sometimes ☐
Guilty	Yes ☐	No ☐	Sometimes ☐
Worried, stressed, tense or anxious	Yes ☐	No ☐	Sometimes ☐
Panicky	Yes ☐	No ☐	Sometimes ☐
Angry or irritable	Yes ☐	No ☐	Sometimes ☐
Ashamed	Yes ☐	No ☐	Sometimes ☐

Other (write in):

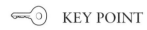

....

....

....

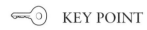 KEY POINT

Emotions are an important and normal part of everyday life. Try to notice changes in how you feel. These changes will often be linked with the thoughts, memories and ideas that are going through your mind at the time. Try to become aware of these thoughts and note them when you have a change in how you feel (your emotions). Try to observe the thoughts as if you were a scientist trying to analyse the problem from a distance.

Summary for area 3: altered feelings/mood in low mood and depression

(?) Having answered the questions above, overall, do I
have problems in this area? Yes ☐ No ☐ Sometimes ☐

Area 4: altered physical sensations/symptoms in depression

In low mood and depression, a person may notice changes in their general wellbeing, with:

- **Altered sleep:** sleep changes commonly occur in depression. This can lead you to feel tired, even after a night in bed. It can be more difficult getting off to sleep, and sometimes sleep is disrupted. Another common change is to awaken in the early hours of the morning and not be able to get off to sleep again.
- **Altered weight:** weight loss can occur as a result of reduced appetite, and weight gain can occur because of comfort eating and reduced activity. For some people, weight gain can cause them to feel even worse.
- **Reduced energy:** low energy levels are a common problem. The person may be tired all the time and feel that they cannot do anything. As a result, in severe depression things that previously would have seemed quite simple, such as getting dressed or washed or going out or playing with the children, may become very difficult.

Other common physical symptoms in depression are:

- **Reduced sex drive:** sex drive is often lost or reduced as part of the general loss of pleasure and interest in things that is normal in depression. Often this is an area the person feels unwilling to talk about, but it may lead to further upset if they are in a relationship. Some antidepressants also cause problems with erections and orgasm (see the workbook *Understanding and using antidepressant medication*).
- **Constipation:** this is common and may be caused by the physical slowing down of the body that occurs in depression. Eating lots of fruit and fibre and drinking a reasonable amount of fluid can help overcome constipation. Increasing activity levels, such as by doing moderate exercise, can also help. Sometimes, constipation is worsened by antidepressants. If you are unsure about this, please discuss it with your doctor.

- **Pain:** if you already have physical problems such as arthritis, depression can make it seem harder to cope. Pain is sometimes an important symptom of depression. Depression may cause tension headaches or contribute to chest or stomach pains, such as those in irritable bowel syndrome.
- **Physical restlessness:** depression can lead to a marked increase in symptoms of physical tension. This may mean that the person finds it difficult to sit still or settle. They may become restless and feel forced to get up and walk around.

The following questions will help you to assess the impact of depression on your own body.

(?) Which physical symptoms have you noticed over the past two weeks?

Wakening earlier than usual	Yes ☐	No ☐	Sometimes ☐
Having difficulty getting off to sleep	Yes ☐	No ☐	Sometimes ☐
Disrupted sleep pattern	Yes ☐	No ☐	Sometimes ☐
Increased/decreased appetite	Yes ☐	No ☐	Sometimes ☐
Increased/decreased weight	Yes ☐	No ☐	Sometimes ☐
Reduced energy	Yes ☐	No ☐	Sometimes ☐
Reduced sex drive	Yes ☐	No ☐	Sometimes ☐
Constipation	Yes ☐	No ☐	Sometimes ☐
Pain	Yes ☐	No ☐	Sometimes ☐
Physical agitation	Yes ☐	No ☐	Sometimes ☐

Other (write in):

✎

....

....

....

Summary for area 4: altered physical sensations/symptoms in depression

(?) Having answered the questions above, overall, do I have problems in this area?　　　　Yes ☐　　No ☐　　Sometimes ☐

You will find some helpful advice about how to tackle a number of physical sensations/symptoms in the workbook *Overcoming sleep problems* (which actually covers more than sleep problems).

The next section will help you to consider the final area – how low mood has affected your behaviour and activity levels.

Section 3   Area 5: altered behaviour in low mood and depression

You have already worked hard in thinking about the first four of the five areas in your five areas assessment – well done! This section moves on to consider the fifth and final area of your five areas assessment – altered behaviour. Some of these changes can make matters worse, but others can help you feel better.

There are several ways in which altered behaviours may worsen feelings of depression. The most common response is to reduce your activity and avoid doing things that seem too difficult. This can worsen how you feel. You may also start to respond in ways that quickly become unhelpful, e.g. drinking alcohol to block out how you feel or choosing to isolate yourself.

The good news is that if you notice these sorts of pattern occurring in your life, then you can begin to make changes to overcome them. Importantly, a whole range of ways in which you respond can be very helpful and boost how you feel. You will find out more about this in the workbook *Helpful and unhelpful things we can do*.

Altered behaviour 1: worsening patterns of reduced activity

When you feel down, it is normal to find it difficult to do things. This is because of:
- Low energy and tiredness ('I'm too tired').
- Low mood and little sense of enjoyment or achievement when things are done.
- Negative thinking and reduced enthusiasm to do things ('I just can't be bothered').

This leads to reduced activity, whereby you reduce or stop doing things **that you value** doing and are important to you.

This leads to:
- Loss of things in life that previously would have given you a sense of fun or achievement, e.g. meeting up with friends, doing hobbies and interests.
- Problems of weakness, stiffness and pain in underused muscles and joints if there is a very large reduction in activity levels.

It can sometimes feel as though everything is too much effort. A pattern of worsening reduced activity may result. This is sometimes called a **vicious circle** or downward spiral. The responses add to the person's problems and worsen how they feel.

You will find out more about reduced activity in the workbook *Overcoming reduced activity and avoidance*. In the meantime, write here any examples of reduced activity you may have noticed:

✎

....

....

....

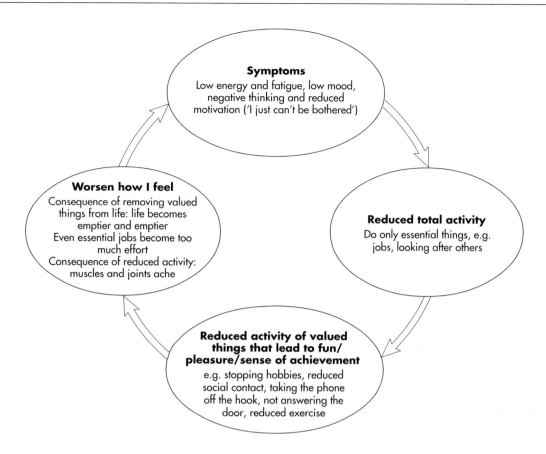

 Does this pattern apply to you?

Have I reduced or stopped doing things I used to enjoy as a result of how I feel?	Yes ☐	No ☐	Sometimes ☐
Has the reduced activity removed things from life that previously gave me a sense of pleasure/achievement?	Yes ☐	No ☐	Sometimes ☐
Has the reduced activity worsened how I feel emotionally or physically?	Yes ☐	No ☐	Sometimes ☐
Overall, has this worsened how I feel?	Yes ☐	No ☐	Sometimes ☐

If you have answered yes or sometimes to all of these questions, then you are experiencing a vicious circle of reduced activity.

The good news is that once you have noticed this is true for you, then you can begin to start working on regaining the pleasurable activities in a planned, step-by-step way. You will find out how to do this in the workbook *Overcoming reduced activity and avoidance*.

Altered behaviour 2: a worsening pattern of avoidance

When somebody becomes anxious, they start to avoid going into places and situations where they predict anxiety will occur. For example, a person with a fear of being in shops will avoid going into large busy shops, someone who has an intense fear of spiders will try to avoid situations where spiders may be present, and someone who experiences high levels of anxiety in social settings will try very hard to avoid such situations.

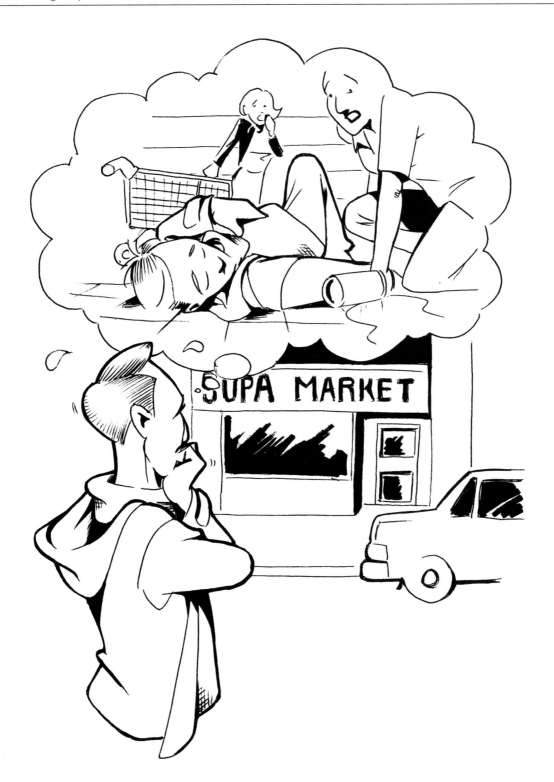

This avoidance adds to the person's problems, because although they may feel less anxious in the short term, in the longer term such actions worsen their problem. A pattern of worsening avoidance may result. This is sometimes called a **vicious circle of avoidance**.

You will find out more about problems of avoidance in the workbook *Overcoming reduced activity and avoidance*. In the meantime, write here any examples of avoidance you may have noticed:

✎

....

....

....

The problem with avoidance is that it teaches you the unhelpful rule that the only way of dealing with a difficult situation is to avoid it. The avoidance also reduces your opportunities to find out that your worst fears do not occur. Avoidance therefore worsens anxiety and further undermines your confidence. This process is summarised in the diagram below.

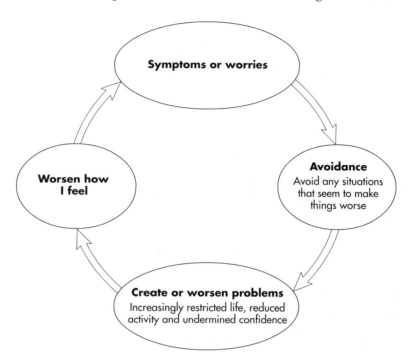

To see whether this pattern applies to you, ask yourself 'What have I stopped or reduced doing because of my worries/concerns?' Remember that at times, avoidance can be quite **subtle**. For example, you might choose to go to the shops at a time when you know they are quiet and then rush through your shopping as quickly as possible.

 Having completed these questions, reflect on your answers using the three questions below:

Am I avoiding things or doing certain actions that are designed to improve how I feel?	Yes ☐	No ☐	Sometimes ☐
Has this reduced my confidence in things and led to an increasingly restricted life?	Yes ☐	No ☐	Sometimes ☐
Overall has this worsened how I feel?	Yes ☐	No ☐	Sometimes ☐

If you have answered yes or sometimes to all three questions, you are experiencing a vicious circle of avoidance.

The good news is that once you have noticed this is true for you, you can start working on tackling any avoidance in a planned, step-by-step way. You will find out how to do this in the workbook *Overcoming reduced activity and avoidance*.

Two final patterns of behaviour commonly occur – one helpful and one unhelpful.

Altered behaviour 3: the pattern of helpful behaviours

When somebody feels low or unwell, it is normal for them to alter what they do in order to try and feel better. Helpful activities may include:

- Talking to friends for support.
- Reading or using self-help materials or attending a self-help group to find out more about the causes and treatment of depression.
- Going to see a doctor or healthcare practitioner to discuss treatments that may be helpful for them.
- Maintaining activities that give pleasure, such as meeting friends.

For people with a spiritual faith, helpful activities may include praying or asking others to pray for you, reading the scriptures and focusing on verses that confirm God's love and support.

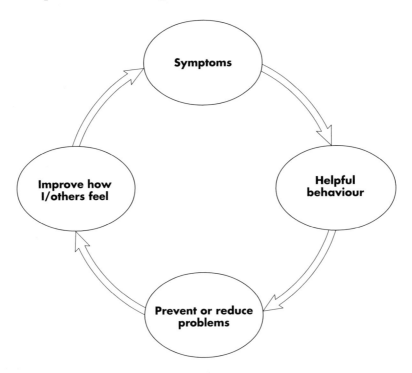

 Having completed these questions, reflect on your answers using the three questions below:

Am I doing any activities or behaviours that improve how I feel?	Yes ☐	No ☐	Sometimes ☐
Are these activities/behaviours definitely helpful in the short- and longer-term for me or for others?	Yes ☐	No ☐	Sometimes ☐
Overall, has this improved how I/others feel?	Yes ☐	No ☐	Sometimes ☐

If you have answered yes or sometimes to all three questions, then you are responding in helpful ways. You should try to build these helpful responses into your life. You will find out more about the ways of building helpful responses in the workbook *Helpful and unhelpful things we can do*.

 LEARNING POINT

Sometimes we think that a behaviour is helpful when in fact it is part of the problem. Typical examples are patterns of excessive drinking and avoidance. Both of these may cause you to feel better in the short term, which is why they can be mistaken as helpful. However, in the medium or long term, they backfire and worsen how you or others feel in some way, whether physically or mentally, or in your relationships. In contrast, a hallmark of a truly helpful activity is that it is good for you and often for others too.

One of the tasks in the section *Putting into practice what you have learned* at the end of this workbook suggests that you write down three things that went well, and why, every day for a week. Stop, think and reflect on this every evening. Try to link this to your responses and use it to identify helpful responses that you can build on in your life.

Altered behaviour 4: the pattern of unhelpful behaviours

Sometimes we try to block how we feel by using unhelpful responses such as:

- Withdrawing into ourselves and cutting ourselves off from our friends.
- Using alcohol to block out how we feel.
- Neglecting ourselves, e.g. by not eating as much as usual.
- Harming ourselves as a way of blocking how we feel, e.g. self-cutting.
- Finding ourselves tempted to do things that we know are unwise or wrong. This might include deliberately taking risks, picking fights or betraying a partner.
- Acting out of frustration or anger to harm or hurt others, e.g. acting in ways to test out the love or support of others. This might include being rude and critical or pushing others away to see how much they really want to support us.

A **pattern of unhelpful behaviour can result.** This is sometimes called a vicious circle or downward spiral. The responses add to the person's problems and worsen how they feel.

You will find out more about unhelpful behaviours in the workbook *Helpful and unhelpful things we can do.* In the meantime, write here any unhelpful behaviours you may have noticed:

✎

....

....

....

Look at the following questions to see whether you have found yourself doing these things in the past week:

Am I responding in ways that are designed to improve how I feel?	Yes ☐	No ☐	Sometimes ☐
Are some of these responses unhelpful in the short or longer term?	Yes ☐	No ☐	Sometimes ☐
Overall, have unhelpful behaviours worsened how I feel?	Yes ☐	No ☐	Sometimes ☐

If you have answered yes or sometimes to all three questions, then you are experiencing a vicious circle of unhelpful behaviour. A key thing to watch out for is how we tend to react to difficult situations in certain ways. By watching out for these patterns, and by choosing to respond differently, we can make large changes in how we feel.

Summary for area 5: altered behaviour in low mood and depression

 Having answered the questions above, overall, do I
have problems in this area?   Yes ☐   No ☐   Sometimes ☐

You will find some helpful advice about how to tackle a number of different altered behaviours in the workbooks *Overcoming reduced activity and avoidance* and *Helpful and unhelpful things we can do.*

You have now finished your five areas assessment. Before you move on, stop for a while and consider what you have learned. How does what you have read help you to make sense of your symptoms?

 How well does this assessment summarise how you feel?

Poorly	Very well
0	10

A summary of how depression has affected you in the past two weeks

The purpose of asking you to carry out the **five areas assessment** is not to demoralise you or to make you feel worse. Instead, by helping you consider how you are now, this can help you plan the areas you need to focus on in order to bring about change. The workbooks in this course can help you begin to tackle each of the five problem areas of depression.

Section 4   The treatments of depression

The main problem areas of low mood and depression are:
- Current situations, relationships or practical problems.
- Altered thinking.
- Altered feelings/mood.
- Altered physical symptoms/bodily sensations.
- Altered behaviour and activity levels, including reduced activity, avoidance and helpful/unhelpful behaviours.

The five areas assessment

You have previously answered questions about each of these five areas. Go back and look at the problems you identified in each area to consider the impact of low mood on you.

Links can occur between each of these areas. Because of this, aiming to **alter any** of these areas may help treat your depression.

KEY POINT

By defining your problems, you have now identified clear targets on which to focus. You can tackle these one step at a time. A key to success is not to throw yourself into tackling everything at once. Slow, steady steps are more likely to result in improvement than starting very enthusiastically and then running out of steam.

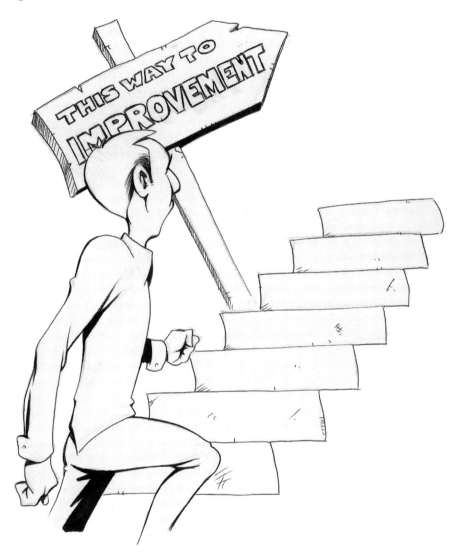

Choosing your targets for change

You may have made all sorts of attempts to change but, unless you have a clear plan and stick to it, change will be very difficult. Planning and selecting the targets to try and change first is a crucial part of successfully moving forwards. By first choosing the areas on which to focus, this also means that you are actively choosing at first **not** to focus on other areas.

Setting yourself targets will help you to focus on how to make the changes needed to get better. To do this, you will need:

- **Short-term targets:** thinking about changes you can make today, tomorrow and next week.
- **Medium-term targets:** changes to be put in place over the next few weeks.
- **Long-term targets:** where you want to be in six months or a year.

The questions that you have answered in this workbook will have helped you to identify the main problem areas that you currently face. The other workbooks can help you to make changes in each of these areas.

The workbooks have been devised to be used either alone or as part of a complete course of workbooks. This workbook is designed to help you to identify your current problem areas. This will help identify which of the other workbooks you need to read. Finally, you can summarise what you have learned and plan how to respond to any future feelings of depression by completing the last workbook *Planning for the future*. This will help you to reduce the chance that depression may affect you like this again.

Course overview: the *Overcoming Depression and Low Mood* course

Starting out: using the course materials . . . and how to keep going if you feel stuck

This workbook provides a brief introduction to low and anxious mood and how the five areas approach can be used to help understand how these affect us. The workbook also focuses on how to use the other workbooks in the course and overcome common blocks to change.

Understanding why I feel as I do

In this workbook, you have learned about how depression alters your thinking and feelings, leading to altered bodily sensations and behaviour. This workbook helps you decide which of these areas you need to focus on changing and helps you decide which of the remaining workbooks you need to read. This is the workbook you are reading now.

Practical problem-solving

In this workbook, you will learn a step-by-step plan that you can use to deal with practical problems, such as debt, housing and problems caused by other people. It will provide you with the tools to tackle any practical problems that you face. This will help you to take more control of your life and the decisions that you make. By feeling more in control of your life, you will improve your confidence in yourself.

Being assertive

Have you ever felt that no one listens to you and that other people seem to walk all over you? Have others commented that they feel that you always walk over them? In this workbook, you will discover how to develop more balanced relationships with others.

Building relationships

How we relate to others can have a strong impact on how we feel. This workbook will help you to rebuild relationships with those around you, helping you to improve damaged relationships and develop new, helpful friendships.

Information for families and friends: how can I offer support?

This workbook is aimed at those around you who you want to inform about the treatment approach. They may be a valuable resource to help you with your problems. Whatever your problem, this workbook will help others reflect on how they can support you.

Noticing and changing extreme and unhelpful thinking

What you think about yourself, others and the situations that occur around you can alter how you feel and affect what you do. This workbook will help you to learn ways of identifying and changing extreme and unhelpful ways of thinking.

Overcoming reduced activity and avoidance

In this workbook, you will learn to change what you do in order to break patterns of worsening reduced activity and avoidance.

Using exercise to boost how you feel

Planned exercise can have really positive impacts on how you feel. This workbook describes how exercise can help, and will help you build some increased activity into your life.

Helpful and unhelpful things we can do

In this workbook, you will learn some effective ways of building helpful responses and at the same time reduce unhelpful behaviours, such as drinking too much alcohol, reassurance-seeking and trying to spend your way out of how you feel.

Alcohol, drugs and you

This short workbook will help you find out about drink and drugs. You will also discover the physical, psychological and social impacts of drinking heavily. The workbook contains some questions to help you work out whether your intake is under control or whether it has become unhelpful and in control of you.

Overcoming sleep problems

Often, when someone is struggling, they not only feel emotionally and mentally low but also notice a range of physical changes. This workbook will help you find out about these common changes and, in particular, will help you to deal with problems of poor sleep and low energy.

Understanding and using antidepressant medication

When someone is depressed, their doctor may suggest they take antidepressant medication. In this workbook, you will find out why doctors suggest this. You will also learn about common fears and concerns that people have when first starting to take antidepressants, so that you can find out for yourself whether antidepressant medication may be helpful for you.

Once you are feeling better, the final workbook of the series can be read to help you summarise what you have learned.

Planning for the future

You will have learned new things about yourself and made changes in how you live your life. This final workbook will help you to identify what you have learned and help you plan for the future. You will create your own personal plan to cope with future problems in your life so that you can face the future with confidence.

Next steps

Look back at your answers to the questions in the last section of this workbook. Then use the following table to help you summarise which workbooks are right for you to read next. You can choose to use any of the workbooks in any order. It is helpful to know, though, that for problems of low mood two of the most effective workbooks are *Practical problem-solving* and *Overcoming reduced activity and avoidance*. If you are taking antidepressants, you may also find it helpful to read the workbook *Understanding and using antidepressant medication* early on.

Workbook	Plan to read	Tick when completed
Starting out	☐	☐
Understanding why I feel as I do	☐	☐
Practical problem-solving	☐	☐
Being assertive	☐	☐
Building relationships	☐	☐
Information for families and friends: how can I offer support?	☐	☐
Noticing and changing extreme and unhelpful thinking	☐	☐
Overcoming reduced activity and avoidance	☐	☐
Using exercise to boost how you feel	☐	☐
Helpful and unhelpful things we can do	☐	☐
Alcohol, drugs and you	☐	☐
Overcoming sleep problems	☐	☐
Understanding and using antidepressant medication	☐	☐
Planning for the future	☐	☐

⚊◯ KEY POINT

In order to change, you will need to choose to try to apply what you will learn **throughout the week,** and not only when you read the workbook or see your healthcare practitioner. The workbooks will encourage you to do this by suggesting tasks for you to carry out in the days after reading each workbook.

These tasks will:
- Help you to put into practice what you have learned in each workbook.
- Gather information so that you can get the most out of the workbook.

Experience has shown that you are likely to make the most progress if you are able to put into practice what you have learned throughout the week.

Workbook summary

In this workbook, you have covered:
- An introduction to low mood, with a chance to complete a timeline of how your problems have developed.
- How to complete your own five areas assessment.
- How to use your own five areas assessment to help you choose which other course workbooks to use.

Putting into practice what you have learned

1 Read through this workbook again and think in detail about how low mood is affecting your thinking, emotional and physical feelings, and behaviour – and what you want to change.

2 Each day for a week, write down **three things** that went well that day. Stop, think and reflect on this each evening. Why did those things go well? Use this to identify any helpful responses that you can build on in your life.

3 Choose **two episodes** over the next week when you feel more upset or depressed. Use the pages that follow this section to **record the impact on your thinking, mood, behaviour and body**. Try to generate a summary of your own depression on each of the five areas of depression (life situation, relationships and practical problems, altered thinking, feelings, physical sensations and behaviour). Look back to the 'Walking down the street' example on page 7 to help you with this task. You will find out more about how to do this in the workbook *Noticing and changing extreme and unhelpful thinking*.

When you have done this, choose your first area to begin working on and slowly read the workbook(s) in that area over a week or two. Put into practice what you have read, and then move on to other areas that you want to cover, making sure you allow yourself time to cover each area before moving on. Try to continue to put into practice what you have learned as you read further workbooks.

(**task**) My practice plan

Write down a clear plan about which workbook you will use next in the practice plan below.

(**?**) What single workbook am I going to use next?

✎
....
....
....

(**?**) **When** am I going to start reading it?

✎
....
....
....

(**?**) **What** problems/difficulties could arise, and how can I overcome these?

✎
....
....
....

Apply the questions for effective change to your plan. Is my planned task:

Useful for understanding or changing how I am?	Yes ☐	No ☐
Specific, so that I will know when I have done it?	Yes ☐	No ☐
Realistic, practical and achievable?	Yes ☐	No ☐
Clear about what I am going to do and when I am going to do it?	Yes ☐	No ☐
An activity that won't be easily blocked or prevented by practical problems?	Yes ☐	No ☐
One that will help me to learn useful things, even if it doesn't work out perfectly?	Yes ☐	No ☐

Try to review your progress in using the workbooks on a weekly basis, and try to make sure the changes are practical and achievable.

If you have difficulties with this workbook, don't worry. Just do what you can.

 A free online training course that supports users of the course is available at www.livinglifetothefull.com. It provides useful additional handouts, teaching sessions and exercises that reinforce and build upon the course workbooks. In addition, you can share ideas and gain encouragement from other readers within a safe, free and moderated discussion forum. You can also sign up for a monthly support bulletin, which will help encourage you to stay on track. Register now for free to find out more.

A request for feedback

An important factor in the development of the five areas assessment workbooks is that the content is updated on a regular basis based upon feedback from users and practitioners. If there are areas within it that you find hard to understand or seem poorly written, please let us know and we will try to improve things in future. Unfortunately, we are unable to provide any specific replies or advice on treatment. To provide feedback, please contact us by:

- *Website:* www.livinglifetothefull.com.
- *Email:* feedback@livinglifetothefull.com.
- *Post:* Dr Chris Williams, Psychological Medicine, Gartnavel Royal Hospital, 1055 Great Western Road, Glasgow G12 0XH.

Acknowledgements

I wish to thank all those who have commented upon this workbook, especially Marie Chellingsworth and Frances Cole.

My notes

....

....

....

....

....

....

....

....

....

....

....

....

....

....

....

....

....

....

....

....

....

....

....

....

....

....

....

....

....

My notes

....

....

A five areas assessment of a specific time when I felt worse

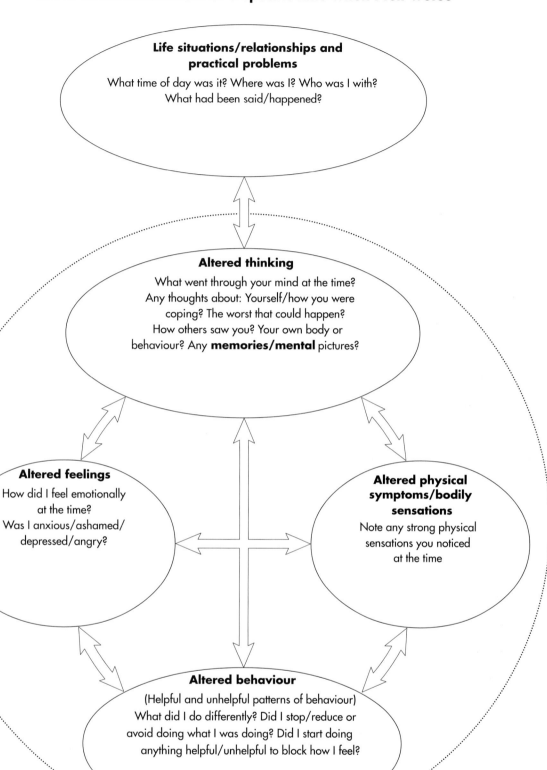

Life situations/relationships and practical problems

What time of day was it? Where was I? Who was I with? What had been said/happened?

Altered thinking

What went through your mind at the time? Any thoughts about: Yourself/how you were coping? The worst that could happen? How others saw you? Your own body or behaviour? Any **memories/mental** pictures?

Altered feelings

How did I feel emotionally at the time? Was I anxious/ashamed/ depressed/angry?

Altered physical symptoms/bodily sensations

Note any strong physical sensations you noticed at the time

Altered behaviour

(Helpful and unhelpful patterns of behaviour) What did I do differently? Did I stop/reduce or avoid doing what I was doing? Did I start doing anything helpful/unhelpful to block how I feel?

Part 2

Making changes

Practical problem-solving

Dr Chris Williams

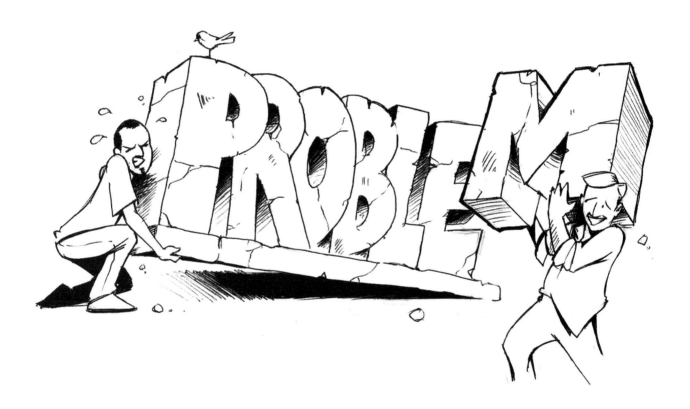

A Five Areas Approach
Helping you to help yourself
www.livinglifetothefull.com

Section *1*   **Introduction**

In this workbook you will:
- Discover how practical problems affect our lives.
- Identify any problems in your own life that can be a target for change.
- See an example of problem-solving in practice and have a chance to apply this to one of your own problems.
- Discover how to make slow, steady changes to your life.
- Plan some next steps to build on this.

Problems and life difficulties can affect us all. Usually, when just one problem arises we can cope. It is when we face a particularly difficult problem or a whole lot of smaller issues arise at the same time that we struggle to cope and feel overwhelmed.

Before you start

Sometimes problems occur because of things we can't control, but sometimes they are the result of things we could have handled differently. For example, problems of debt may build up because we have ignored the problem or kept spending at far too high a level without bearing in mind our income. Perhaps we have not responded in ways that would have prevented things worsening at an earlier stage.

Think about your behaviour

Do you notice the same sorts of problems occurring again? If so, is there anything that you keep doing (or not doing) that leads to the problem? If so, using the workbook *Helpful and unhelpful things we can do* may be useful.

Think about your thinking

Before starting out to tackle your practical problems, it is important to choose the right target. The very first thing to do is to consider whether the problem really is such an issue. Is it possible that things are being blown up out of all proportion because of how you feel at the moment? If so, then the workbook *Noticing and changing extreme and unhelpful thinking* can help you get things back into perspective.

Overview

By working through the seven steps outlined in this workbook, you will learn an approach that enables you to solve your own problems.

The steps of problem-solving include:
- Approaching each problem separately and in turn.
- Defining the problem clearly.
- Breaking down seemingly enormous and unmanageable problems into smaller parts that are then easier to solve. By approaching your practical problems one step at a time, it is possible to begin tackling them.

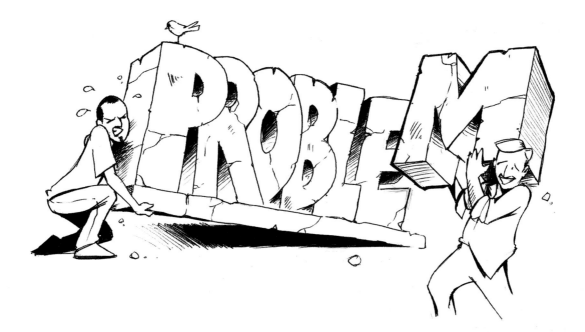

Think about these questions:

(?) What might be the advantage of planning to change just one problem at first?

✎

....

....

....

(?) What are the potential dangers of trying to change everything at once?

✎

....

....

....

Section 2 The seven steps to problem-solving: Paul's example

Step 1: identify and clearly define the problem as precisely as possible

 EXAMPLE

Paul's problem

Paul has been unwell for a number of months and is off work and not earning. He has identified his general problem as being 'I have difficulties with money worries or debts'.

Is this a good first target? Paul answers the next question to think about this further:

  Is this a small, focused problem I can tackle in one step?   Yes ☐   No ☑

Paul needs to break down the problem into some **smaller steps** that he can tackle first. These will all add up to help him slowly sort out his larger problem with money worries.

One way of thinking about this process is to think of it as a **funnelling process** – funnelling down from the general problem area to a more specific problem that you tackle first.

The funnel process: defining a specific problem

General problem: *'I don't have enough money'*

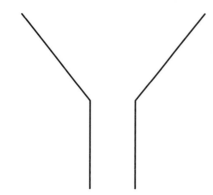

Specific problem: *'I can't pay my credit-card bill this month'*

 EXAMPLE

Breaking down the problem into smaller parts

To identify a better first target, Paul answers the question 'Exactly what aspect of not having enough money is causing me a problem at the moment?' By answering this question, he is able to define more clearly the problem he wants to tackle first as: 'I can't pay my credit-card bill this month.'

Is this a small, focused problem I can tackle in one step?　　　　Yes ☑　No ☐

This is a good first target to tackle. Although there may be a single solution (e.g. recover quickly, get back to work, inherit some money, or win the lottery), often these solutions are unlikely to happen (e.g. winning the lottery) or may not happen as soon as he wishes (e.g. getting back to work). Paul therefore needs to think about a smaller target that can be achieved quickly and will make a helpful impact on his money problems. Here, sorting out his credit-card bill won't solve all his financial problems, but it may be a useful first step. This should be small enough to be possible, but big enough to move him forwards.

Step 2: think up as many solutions as possible to achieve your initial goal

One problem that people often face when they feel overwhelmed by practical problems is that they cannot see a way out. It can seem difficult to even start tackling the difficulty. One way around this is to try to step back from the problem and see whether any other solutions are possible. This approach is called **brainstorming**. The more solutions that are generated, the more likely a good solution will emerge. The purpose of brainstorming is to come up with as many ideas as possible. From these ideas, you hope to be able to identity a realistic, practical and achievable solution towards overcoming your problem.

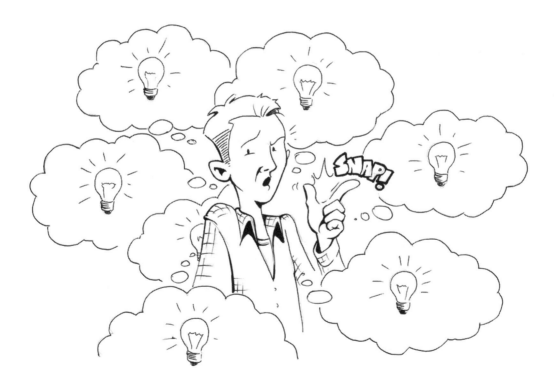

EXAMPLE

Paul's problem

Possible options, including some ridiculous ideas at first, are:

● Ignore the problem completely: it may go away.

● Mug someone or rob a bank.

● Try to arrange a loan or overdraft from the bank and use this to pay off the bill.

● Pay off a very small part of the money (the minimum asked for).

● Switch my credit-card payments to another credit card with a lower interest rate.

● Speak to a counsellor with skills in debt repayments.

● Speak to the credit-card company to see whether it will agree different repayment terms.

Step 3: look at the advantages and disadvantages of each possible solution

Suggestion	Advantage	Disadvantage
Ignore the problem completely	Easier in the short term, and with no embarrassment	The problems will worsen in the long term; it will still have to be tackled at some time
Mug someone or rob a bank	It would get me some money	It's unethical and wrong. I couldn't do it. I might be arrested. I couldn't harm someone else in this way. That's just ridiculous
Arrange a loan or overdraft	It would allow me a better rate of interest than paying off the high rate on my credit card. I could also spread the payments over a longer time. I have a good banking record so it's likely to work and be quite fast as well	How would I do this? It would be scary seeing the bank manager. I may be wrong about whether they think I'm a good credit risk. They may say no
Pay off the minimum payment	Good short-term answer. It would prevent me defaulting on the payments	The debt wouldn't get any smaller, and the interest rates will make it larger and larger. I'll never be able to pay it off
Switch to a cheaper credit card	This would be a lot cheaper. There are lots of good deals around, with cheaper introductory rates	I would need to look at the small print of the different agreements and complete all the paperwork
Speak to a debt counsellor	I hear they can be very good	I'd feel embarrassed talking to them. How do you contact them?

Suggestion	Advantage	Disadvantage
Inform the credit-card company and ask for different repayment terms	It would provide the company with clear information. It's in their best interests for me to keep up the payments. They may be flexible and allow a repayment break at lower interest	It seems quite scary to do this

Step 4: choose one of the solutions

The chosen solution should be an option that will make a sensible first step in achieving your goal. It should be realistic and likely to succeed. The decision needs to be based on all the answers to Step 3.

 EXAMPLE

Paul's choice

Paul decides, on balance, to arrange a bank loan or overdraft. Other suggestions might also have worked, but this suggestion seems a reasonable solution for him based on his previous record with the bank. If he had had a poorer bank record, then choosing one of the other options would have been better.

The solution should be an option that fulfils the following criteria:

Will it be useful for changing how you are?	Yes ✔	No ☐
Is it a clear task, so that you will know when you have done it?	Yes ✔	No ☐
Is it something that is realistic, practical and achievable?	Yes ✔	No ☐

Step 5: plan the steps needed to carry out the solution

 EXAMPLE

Paul's plan

I could phone my bank. I have the phone number on my bank statement. I'm quite nervous, so I'm going to plan out what I am going to say in advance. I will phone up and ask to arrange a time to come in. I will tell them I am having problems repaying my credit card because I am off work sick. I will ask whether I can come in to see someone in the afternoon because I feel better then. I think it's best if I also phone them in the afternoon. I'm more likely to get straight through to them then, and also I generally feel more confident after lunch.

Paul makes sure that, as part of his plan, he builds in some thought on what helpful things he could do if his plan does not succeed fully.

Next, Paul needs to apply the questions for effective change to his plan, to check how practical and achievable it is.

The questions for effective change

Is the planned solution one that:

Will be useful for understanding or changing how I am?	Yes ✓	No ☐
Is a specific task, so that I will know when I have done it?	Yes ✓	No ☐
Is realistic, practical and achievable?	Yes ✓	No ☐
Makes clear what I am going to do and when I am going to do it?	Yes ✓	No ☐
Is an activity that won't be easily blocked or prevented by practical problems?	Yes ✓	No ☐
Will help me to learn useful things, even if it doesn't work out perfectly?	Yes ✓	No ☐

Paul can answer yes to each of the questions. If he couldn't, then he would need to think what changes he could make in order to alter or improve his plan.

Note: part of this planning phase should include Paul having a planned response of how to react if his request is turned down.

What if it doesn't work out?

Paul writes out his plan:

'If it doesn't work out I'll be definitely disappointed. I'll need to react quickly to pay off the minimum on the card so I don't get a penalty charge. After that I'll go back to my list of brainstorming tasks. I'll get in touch with a debt counsellor at the Citizens' Advice Bureau and ask their advice.'

Step 6: carry out the plan

Paul telephones the bank that afternoon as planned. Just before he does this, he feels quite scared. He predicts that the company representative 'will humiliate me and turn down my request'. He records how much he believed this at the time, from 0% (not believing it at all) to 100% (believing it fully). At the time, he believes this 75%. He also records how anxious he feels at the time, from 0% (no anxiety at all) to 100% (maximum anxiety possible). Overall, he felt about 70% anxious before he phoned.

Paul decides to challenge these fears and phones the company anyway. When he phones, the line is engaged. He tries again two minutes later. The phone is answered by an electronic answering service, which asks him to choose a service from five options. Paul is surprised by this and is quite taken aback. He becomes flustered and immediately puts down the phone.

His immediate thought is 'What an idiot! I should be able to do this.' Over the next few minutes, he is able to challenge this thought. He remembers that this sort of thing happens a lot with banks. He just needs to be ready for it next time. He decides to learn from what happened and tries again. He phones again but plans to have a pen and paper available to write down the different options. He finds that the current option for those with payment difficulties is option 2. He selects this and arranges an appointment. He finds that as he talks to the person on the phone, they are polite and friendly. His anxiety begins to drop and his belief in his thought that they 'will humiliate me and turn down my request' drops from 75% to only 30% by the end of the conversation.

Two days later, when he goes to the bank, he begins to feel quite scared again. He rates himself as 80% anxious and feels physically tense and on edge. He predicts: 'The manager will humiliate me and turn down my request.' He also worries that the credit-card company will then demand immediate payment and issue a court summons. He believes these negative predictions about 90% at the time. Paul is almost convinced he will be rejected. Importantly, again Paul plucks up his courage and decides to challenge these fears and go to the bank anyway. This is the best way to experiment and test out how true our fears are – by acting against them and seeing what happens.

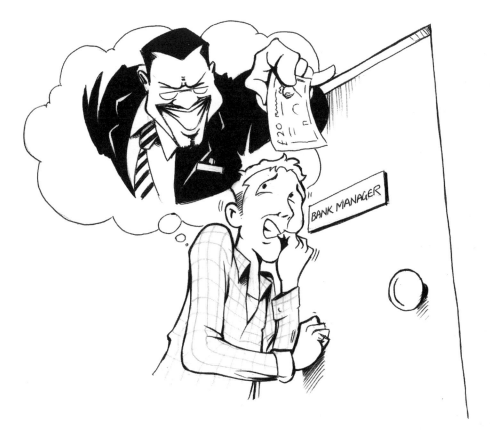

When he arrives at the bank, Paul is surprised to be met by a friendly bank assistant rather than the manager. She says that she is his personal account manager. She offers Paul a cup of tea, and they talk in a office so that their discussion is confidential. She tells him that this is a common problem. Because he has banked with them for several years and has a good banking record, she says there will be no problems in offering him a loan at a preferential rate. Paul agrees, and is happy with how things went. His fears were not correct. He was offered a loan, and at a rate that he can afford.

As Paul leaves the interview, he re-rates his anxiety during and after the interview. It has dropped from 80% before the interview, to 50% during the interview, to nearly nothing afterwards. In fact he feels very positive. His belief that he would be humiliated and end up being taken to court has also dropped from 90%, to 50% during the interview, and then to zero afterwards. Again, by facing his fears, he has been able to challenge them.

Step 7: review the outcome

Was the selected solution successful?	Yes ✓	No ☐
Did it help pay off the credit-card debt (the target problem)?	Yes ✓	No ☐
Were there any disadvantages to using this approach?	Yes ✓	No ☐

What have I learned from doing this?

> 'Things went smoothly the second time I phoned up. Even when the problem arose when I hung up on the first occasion, I learned from it and didn't give up. I altered my plan by getting the pen and paper. By phoning back and not giving up, I sorted out my problem and also realised that my worries were quite wrong.'

In this case, Paul's plan went smoothly. Even if there were any problems, he could have learned from them and used them to improve his next attempt to solve the problem.

The example used shows how the technique might be applied to this situation. However, it also works for any day-to-day difficulties.

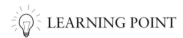 LEARNING POINT

Paul chose the option of going to his bank because he knew previously he had a good banking record. If he hadn't had a good record, then he wouldn't have chosen this response. Even so, sometimes we can all overestimate how likely something is to succeed. If Paul had been turned down for the loan, he would have been surprised and upset. He had, however, already created a plan (at step 5) of what he could do if he was turned down. And even if he had been turned down, he would have learned some things.

For example, even if Paul was turned down, he would have achieved the following:
- He has a clear idea of the target problem to work on.
- He has a list of alternative options he could use to tackle the problem. Some of these may well be effective.
- He has learned an approach he can try again.
- He has realised that his worrying thoughts are not always accurate. For example, he was not humiliated when he phoned the bank or at the interview. He has also learned that facing up to his fears causes his anxiety to drop.
- He can take what he has learned and include it in his own review.

You now have the option of practising this approach.

Section *3* My problem-solving

Think about how you can begin to tackle the problems you face in your own life. Remember that the aim isn't to change things across the board. Instead, the plan is to tackle specific problems.

Step 1: identify and clearly define the problem as precisely as possible

You probably already have a clear idea of the range of problems you are facing. Remember that we are talking here about problems with other people, housing, job, lack of job, etc. This workbook addresses how to tackle **external problems** rather than inner issues such as problematic thinking and emotions.

The important first step to problem-solving is to make sure that you have identified a single, focused target problem. This involves defining the problem you are going to tackle. This step is particularly important if you feel overwhelmed by a wide range of different problems.

(?) The following checklist can help you identify a problem area that you want to tackle:

I have relationship difficulties, such as arguments	Yes ☐	No ☐	Sometimes ☐
My relatives don't really talk to me or offer me any support	Yes ☐	No ☐	Sometimes ☐
There is no one around who I can really talk to	Yes ☐	No ☐	Sometimes ☐
There are things that others close to me are doing/not doing that create or worsen my problems	Yes ☐	No ☐	Sometimes ☐
I have difficulties with money worries or debt	Yes ☐	No ☐	Sometimes ☐
I don't like where I live	Yes ☐	No ☐	Sometimes ☐
I am having problems with my neighbours	Yes ☐	No ☐	Sometimes ☐
I don't enjoy my job	Yes ☐	No ☐	Sometimes ☐

Other problems:

....

....

....

Make sure this is an **external problem**, for example with other people, housing or money, rather than a problem with your own thoughts or emotions.

Look back at your list and from this identify a single initial target area that you will focus on. This is particularly important if you have ticked a number of boxes in the checklist. It is not possible to overcome all these areas at once. Instead, you need to choose one area on which to focus to start with.

Write down one problem area you want to work on here:

✎

....

....

....

Remember that this should be an external problem rather than an issue to do with your own thoughts or emotions.

It may be that the thought of making changes here seems daunting or impossible. The key is to use a **step-by-step** approach where no step seems too large. This first step needs to be something that gets you moving in the right direction.

Ask yourself whether you need to break down this problem area into a number of smaller, more achievable targets. You can do this by funnelling down from a general problem area to a more specific problem you can tackle first. Look at Paul's example on pages 6–7 if in doubt.

Ask yourself whether this is a good first target.

(?) Is this a small, focused problem that I can tackle in one step?   Yes ☐   No ☐

(✿) CHOICE POINT

If you answer yes, then skip to Step 2. If you answer no, then keep reading about how to identify a realistic first target.

(!) IMPORTANT POINT

Reality check: is this a realistic target for change?

Imagine if throughout your entire life a particular relative has been difficult with you. It is probably unrealistic that your plan should include them changing to suddenly be really easy to get on with. Instead, you could focus on planning how to live with them as they are. If they do change that's great, but we have to be realistic that any change they make might be quite small and take some time.

Funnelling down: choosing a clear first step on which to work

What smaller steps do you need to tackle first? Select a smaller aspect of the problem that you wish to change at the present time. Write it here:

✎

....

....

....

Again, remember that this should be an external problem, and not an issue to do with your own thoughts or emotions.

(?) Is this a clear, focused problem?   Yes ☐   No ☐

(?) Is it realistic, practical and achievable?   Yes ☐   No ☐

If you answer no to either question, then rewrite your target problem here:

✎

....

....

....

Step 2: think up as many solutions as possible to achieve your initial goal

The purpose of brainstorming is to try to come up with as many ideas as possible. Among these ideas, you hope to be able to identity a realistic, practical and achievable solution. Completely wacky ideas should be included as well, even if you would never choose them in practice. This can help you adopt a flexible approach to the problem.

Try to **think broadly**. Useful questions to help you to think up possible solutions might include:

- What advice would you give a friend who was trying to tackle the same problem? Sometimes we can think of solutions for others more easily than for ourselves.
- What ridiculous solutions can I include as well as more sensible ones?
- What helpful suggestions would others (e.g. family, friends, work colleagues) make?
- How could you look at the solutions facing you differently? For example, what would you have said before you felt like this, or what might you say about the situation say in five years' time?
- What approaches have you tried in the past in similar circumstances?

If you feel stuck, sometimes doing this task with someone you trust can be helpful.

Brainstorming my problem

Write down your ideas, including ridiculous options:

✎

....

....

....

....

....

....

....

....

....

....

....

Step 3: look at the advantages and disadvantages of each possible solution

The next step is to think about the pros and cons of each possible option.

My suggestion	Advantage	Disadvantage

What you are looking for is a **step-by-step approach** in which no step seems too large. The sort of solution you are looking for is, therefore, something that gets you moving in the right direction. This should be small enough to be possible, but big enough to move you forwards.

Step 4: choose one of the solutions

The chosen solution should be an option that will make a sensible solution in tackling your problem. It should be realistic and likely to succeed. The decision needs to be based on all your answers to Step 3.

Look at your own responses in Step 3. From this, you should choose a solution. Write your preferred solution here:

....

....

....

This solution should be an option that fulfils the following criteria:

Will it be **useful** for changing how you are?	Yes ☐	No ☐
Is it a **clear** task, so that you will know when you have done it?	Yes ☐	No ☐
Is it something that is **realistic**, practical and achievable?	Yes ☐	No ☐

Step 5: plan the steps needed to carry it out

🔑 KEY POINT

You need to generate a clear plan that will help you to decide exactly **what** you are going to do and **when** you are going to do it. It is useful to **write down** the steps needed to carry out your solution. This will help you to plan what to do and allows you to predict possible problems that might arise. Remember to build into your plan some thought about what you will do if the plan doesn't succeed fully.

My plan

Include ways of tackling any possible blocks that might get in the way.

✎

....

....

....

....

....

....

....

....

....

....

....

....

....

....

....

....

....

....

....

This is the key part of the problem-solving process. Be as precise as possible in your plan. Next, apply the questions for effective change to your plan to check how practical and achievable it is.

Is my planned task one that:

	Yes	No
Will be useful for understanding or changing how I am?	☐	☐
Is a specific task, so that I will know when I have done it?	☐	☐
Is realistic, practical and achievable?	☐	☐
Makes clear what I am going to do and when I am going to do it?	☐	☐
Is an activity that won't be easily blocked or prevented by practical problems?	☐	☐
Will help me to learn useful things, even if it doesn't work out perfectly?	☐	☐

You should be able to answer yes to each of these questions. If your current plan has failed on one of the questions, try to change or alter things so that any poorly planned aspects are improved.

Part of this planning phase should include planning what you will do if your initial plan doesn't work out fully.

What if it doesn't work out? Write your plan of what you can do next here:

✎

....

....

....

Step 6: carry out the plan

Pay attention to your thoughts about what will happen before, during and after you have completed your plan. If this seems too difficult, then skip straight to step 7.

(task) Write down any extreme and unhelpful thoughts you noticed. Record how much you believed them at the time, from 0% (not at all) to 100% (fully).

My thoughts:

✎

....

....

....

I believed this   % before the task.

I believed this   % during the task.

I believed this   % after the task.

(task) Record how anxious you felt at the time, from 0% (no anxiety at all) to 100% (maximum possible anxiety).

My level of anxiety was   % before the task.

My level of anxiety was   % during the task.

My level of anxiety was   % after the task.

Remember that as you carry out the plan you are undermining your old fears by acting against them.

Step 7: review the outcome

Write what happened here:

....

....

....

....

....

....

....

....

....

....

....

....

....

....

....

....

....

....

....

Was the approach successful?	Yes ☐	No ☐
Did it help to improve things?	Yes ☐	No ☐
Were there any disadvantages to using this approach?	Yes ☐	No ☐

(?) What have I learned from doing this? Write down any helpful lessons or information you have learned from what happened. If things didn't go quite as you hoped, try to learn from this. How could you make things different during your next attempt to tackle the problem?

✎

....

....

....

....

....

....

....

....

....

....

....

....

....

....

....

....

....

....

....

....

....

If you noticed problems with your plan

Choosing realistic targets for change is important. Were you too ambitious or unrealistic in choosing your target? Sometimes a problem-solving approach may be blocked by something happening unexpectedly. Perhaps something didn't happen as you planned or someone reacted in an unexpected way. Try to learn from what happened.

(?) If you noticed a problem with your plan, how could you change how you approach the problem to help you create a realistic action plan?

✎

....

....

....

....

....

....

....

....

....

....

....

....

....

Putting into practice what you have learned

Choose only one or two problems and use the seven-step problem-solving approach during the next few days.

After a week or so of trying this, read the final part of the workbook.

Section 4 Planning the next steps

Now that you have considered how your first planned activity went, the next step is to plan another activity to build on this. You need to think about your **short-**, **medium-** and **longer-term** targets. Did your problem-solving plan help you to solve the problem completely? You may need to plan out other solutions in order to tackle different aspects of your problem. The key is to build one step upon another.

For example, Paul's last plan helped him deal with the immediate issue (needing to pay his credit card this month). His loan will have helped tide things over for a time. However, there are other issues that he also needs to address, such as reducing his spending while he's not working and looking at ways of getting back to work.

Steps should always be realistic, practical and achievable. Without this sort of step-by-step approach, you may find that although you take some steps forward, these are all in different directions and you lose your focus and motivation. Use what you have learned to build on what you did.

Many people find this approach takes quite a lot of practice. It may be tempting to be too ambitious and try to sort out everything all at once. Remember: large changes can be achieved by moving one step at a time. Making slow, sure steps will also boost your confidence and increase your sense of having the ability to deal with the problems you face.

Do:
- Continue to plan to alter only one problem area at a time.
- Break down the problem into smaller parts, each of which builds towards your eventual goal. There can be as many or as few steps as you want in your plan.
- Produce a plan to slowly tackle the wider problem in an effective way.
- Be realistic in your goals.
- Use the *Questions for effective change* on page 18 to help you plan each step.
- Write down your plan in detail so that you will be able to put it into practice this week.

Don't:
- Choose too ambitious a target to do next.
- Try to alter too many areas of your life all at once.
- Be negative and think 'Nothing can be done'. (Instead, try to experiment to find out whether this negative thinking is true or helpful.)

Most difficulties can be overcome using this approach. Remember that the main reason why a plan might be ineffective is if you don't allow yourself to believe that change is possible.

Once you have chosen the next step you wish to change, write it down here.
My next target is:

....

....

....

Use the steps in Section 3 of this workbook to create your plan. These are also summarised in shorter form as an example and as a worksheet in the final two pages of this workbook.

Workbook summary

In this workbook, you have:
- Discovered how practical problems affect our lives.
- Identified any problems in your own life that can be a target for change.
- Seen an example of problem-solving in practice and had a chance to apply this to one of your own problems.
- Discovered how to make slow, steady changes to your life.
- Planned some next steps to build on this.

Putting into practice what you have learned

Continue to put into practice what you have learned over the next few weeks. Do not try to solve all your problems at once. Plan out what to do at a pace that is right for you. Build changes one step at a time. Use the blank summary sheet at the end of this workbook to help you plan these changes. If you are stuck or unsure what to do, discuss this with a friend or your healthcare practitioner.

My notes

....

....

....

....

....

....

....

....

....

....

....

....

....

....

....

....

....

....

....

....

....

....

....

....

....

....

....

....

My notes

....

....

The seven steps to practical problem-solving: Paul's example

By working through the seven steps below, you can learn an approach that enables you to solve your own problems.

Example

Paul is off work sick and has a problem: 'I don't have enough money.' A more specific way to identify the problem would be for Paul to ask himself: 'Exactly what aspect of not having enough money is causing me a problem at the moment?' By answering this, Paul is able to define more clearly the problem he wants to tackle first: 'I can't pay my credit-card bill this month.'

Step 1: identify and clearly define the problem as precisely as possible

Example: I don't have any money – so I am not able to pay my credit-card bill this month.

Step 2: think up as many solutions as possible to achieve your initial goal

Example: Ignore the problem. Rob a bank. Arrange a bank loan. Pay off the minimum amount asked for. Switch to a lower-rate credit card. Speak to a debt counsellor. Speak to the credit-card company to try and agree different repayment terms.

Step 3: look at the advantages and disadvantages of each possible solution

Example: Ignore it: advantages – easier in the short term; disadvantages – problems will worsen.

Step 4: choose one of the solutions

Example: The solution should be an option that is useful, clear and realistic.

Step 5: plan the steps needed to carry out the solution

Example: Decide to phone the bank in the afternoon when feeling well. Find the phone number on a bank statement. Explain that I am off work sick. Ask for an afternoon appointment as I often feel ill in the morning. Is it an activity that: Will be useful for understanding or changing how I am? Is a specific task, so that I will know when I have done it? Is realistic, practical and achievable? Makes clear what I am going to do and when I am going to do it? Is an activity that won't be easily blocked or prevented by practical problems? Will help me to learn useful things even if it doesn't work out perfectly?

Step 6: carry out the plan

Example: If you do not succeed with your plan first time, do not be put off. Record and rate (0–100%) your thoughts and your level of anxiety before, during and after you do this. The best way to challenge fears is to act against them.

Step 7: review the outcome

Example: Was the selected solution successful? Did it help pay off the credit-card bill? Were there any disadvantages? What have you learned from the situation? How can you put what you have learned into practice?

Practical problem-solving worksheet

Step 1: identify and clearly define the problem as precisely as possible

Select the problem area you will tackle:

✎

....

....

Do you need to break down the problem into smaller targets that are more practical, realistic and achievable in the next week or so? If so, write your new target here:

✎

....

....

Step 2: think up as many solutions as possible to achieve your initial goal

Brainstorm: what advice would you give a friend? Include ridiculous ideas as well. What have others said? What would you say in five years' time?

✎

....

....

....

Step 3: look at the advantages and disadvantages of each possible solution

Use another sheet of paper to do this.

Step 4: choose one of the solutions

Base this on your answers in Step 3. The solution should be an option that is useful, clear and realistic.

Step 5: plan the steps needed to carry out the solution

Use another sheet of paper to plan the steps.

Use the questions for effective change to check how well planned the activity is. Is it an activity that: Will be useful for understanding or changing how I am? Is a specific task, so that I will know when I have done it? Is realistic, practical and achievable? Makes clear what I am going to do and when I am going to do it? Won't be easily blocked or prevented by practical problems? Will help me to learn useful things even if it doesn't work out perfectly?

Include a plan of what you will do if your solution doesn't work out fully.

Step 6: carry out the plan

Record and rate (0–100%) your thoughts and worries and your level of anxiety before, during and after you do this. Remember that the best way to challenge fears is to act against them.

Step 7: review the outcome

Was the selected solution successful? Where there any disadvantages? What have you learned from the situation? How can you put what you have learned into practice?

Use another sheet of paper to plan the steps.

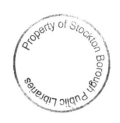

Being assertive

Dr Chris Williams

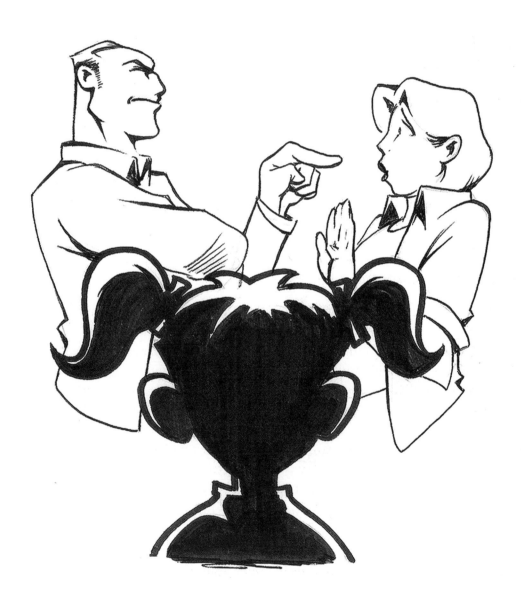

A Five Areas Approach
Helping you to help yourself
www.livinglifetothefull.com

Section 1   **Introduction**

In this workbook you will:
- Discover the differences between passive, aggressive, passive-aggressive and assertive styles of behaviour.
- Learn the rules of assertion and how you can put them into practice in everyday situations.
- Practise assertive techniques in your own life.
- Review your own style of communicating with others.

What is assertiveness?

Assertiveness is being able to stand up for yourself, making sure your opinions and feelings are considered, and not letting other people always get their way. It is **not** the same as aggressiveness. You can be assertive without being forceful or rude. Instead, assertiveness is stating clearly what you expect and insisting that your rights are considered.

Assertion is a skill that can be learned. It is a way of communicating and behaving with others that helps the person to become more confident and aware of themselves and their own needs as an individual, rather than as a partner, friend, parent, etc.

Each of us at some time in our lives, however confident we are, will find it difficult to deal with certain situations we encounter. Examples of such situations could be:
- Dealing with unhelpful shop assistants.
- Asking someone to return something they have borrowed.
- Reacting to angry colleagues at work.
- Communicating our feelings to a partner, family member or friend.
- Saying no to other people's demands.

Often in life we deal with these situations by losing our temper, by saying nothing or by giving in. This may leave us feeling unhappy, angry or out of control and may not actually solve the problem. This tendency to react in either an unassertive or an aggressive way may become even more of a problem if we are struggling with low mood or anxiety. These problems cause a loss of confidence and self-worth, which makes us more likely to give in to everyone around us. Sometimes the reverse happens and we dig in our heels and become very irritable towards everyone else.

Where does assertiveness come from?

As we grow up, we learn patterns of how to relate to others as a result of the things that happen to us. We model ourselves upon those around us, including our parents, teachers and friends, and other influences such as television and magazines. Sometimes our self-confidence is eroded, for example through being bullied or ridiculed at school or criticised within the family. This can make us more likely to react passively or aggressively in our adult lives.

The good news is that although we may have learned to react passively or aggressively in life, we can learn to become more assertive by using assertiveness skills.

Let's first look at the effects of acting in a **passive** or an **aggressive** way, and then contrast this with the impact of assertion.

The key elements of passive behaviour

Passive behaviour describes a situation where we always say yes. We don't express our feelings, needs, rights and opinions. Instead, we always choose others' needs over our own.

- **Feelings:** we bottle up our own feelings or express them in indirect or unhelpful ways.
- **Needs:** we see the other person's needs as more important than our own. We give in to them all the time.
- **Rights:** the other person has rights, but we do not apply the same rights to ourselves.
- **Opinions:** we see ourselves as having little or nothing to contribute. The other person is always right. We may be frightened to say what we think.

The aim of passive behaviour is to **avoid conflict** at all times and to **please others**. It is usually driven by a fear of not wanting to upset others or be disliked by others.

Short-term effects of passive behaviour

- We feel less tense – at least for a while.
- We avoid feeling guilty.

Long-term effects of passive behaviour

- Loss of self-esteem.
- Increased tensions, leading to stress, anger and depression.

The result is that in the longer term, we feel worse. Our passive behaviour also causes others to become irritated and to develop a lack of respect for us. Others may take us for granted and increasingly expect us to drop everything to help them.

The key elements of aggressive behaviour

Aggression is the opposite of assertion. Aggression occurs when we express our own feelings, needs, rights and opinions with no respect for other people.

- **Feelings:** we express our feelings in a demanding, angry and inappropriate way.
- **Needs:** we see our own needs as being more important than others' needs. Others' needs are ignored or dismissed.
- **Rights:** we aggressively stand up for our own rights, but do so in such a way that we violate the rights of other people.
- **Opinions:** we see ourselves as having something to contribute. In contrast, we see other people as having little or nothing to contribute.

The aim of aggression is to win, even at the expense of others. Try to think of a time when someone else has been aggressive to you and ignored your opinions. How did it make you feel about them and yourself?

Aggression has both short-term and long-term consequences.

Short-term effects of aggressive behaviour

- We win and get our own way.
- We feel less angry or tense.
- We feel more powerful and in control.

Long-term effects of aggressive behaviour

- We may feel guilty or ashamed.
- Our self-confidence and self-esteem can worsen because we realise we are doing things poorly.
- We damage our relationships and cause resentment in those around us. We can end up isolated with few friends.

Overall, the longer-lasting effects of using aggression cause problems for the person and for those around them.

Passive aggression (indirect aggression)

Sometimes people mix elements of aggressive and passive responses to create a more indirect form of aggression. This is sometimes referred to as **passive aggression** or **indirect aggression**. In indirect aggression, the person shows their displeasure in indirect ways. Rather than being openly critical, everything is done in a hidden and indirect way. For example, they may stare or raise their eyebrows questioningly when they disagree with what someone is doing or saying. Instead of saying openly and assertively that they disagree, they avoid saying anything directly and instead show their disapproval indirectly, for example by screwing up their face in a dismissive manner or looking around as if bored while the other person is speaking.

People who do this often need to be in control but also want to be liked. They often feel angry but don't show it directly – hence, the description of this type of behaviour as **passive-aggressive behaviour** or **indirect aggression**. Their behaviour is usually driven by low self-esteem and a deep-seated fear that means they always have to be seen as competent. They may manipulate people to get their own way rather than openly asking for what they want. Although they may appear to think highly of others, there is often an undercurrent of disapproval. People relating to someone who is indirectly aggressive often feel confused and frustrated. Typically, the person who is indirectly aggressive denies their true feelings and blames others for any relationship or communication difficulties. Their main weapon is guilt, and they know exactly how to create guilt in those around them. This is especially difficult for those around them who have a strong desire to be liked. They perceive a problem in the relationship, but everything is denied and they feel that they are being blamed.

Regardless of whether there are issues of aggression, indirect aggression or passivity, there is a cure – assertive communication.

The key elements of assertive behaviour

Assertion is expressing our own feelings, needs, rights and opinions while maintaining respect for other people.

- **Feelings:** when we are being assertive, we are able to express our feelings in a direct, honest and appropriate way.
- **Needs:** we have needs that have to be met, otherwise we feel undervalued, rejected, angry or sad.
- **Rights:** we all have basic human rights and it is possible to stand up for your own rights in such a way that does not violate another person's rights.
- **Opinions:** we have something to contribute, irrespective of other people's views.

Assertion is not about winning. It is concerned with being able to walk away feeling that we put across what we wanted to say.

(?) Try to think about a time when someone else has been assertive with you and respected your opinion. How did you feel about them and yourself?

About me, I felt:

....

....

....

About them, I felt:

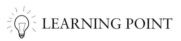

....

....

....

The benefits of assertion

Assertiveness is an **attitude** towards yourself and others that is helpful and honest. In assertiveness, we ask for what we want:

- Directly and openly.
- Appropriately, respecting your own opinions and rights and expecting others to do the same.
- Confidently, and without undue anxiety.

In assertiveness, we try not to:

- Violate people's rights.
- Expect other people to know, magically, what we want.
- Freeze with anxiety and avoid difficult issues.

The result is improved self-confidence and mutual respect from others.

LEARNING POINT

The rules of assertion

The following rules provide you with 12 principles that can help you live your life more assertively.
I have the right to:

1 Respect myself, who I am and what I do.
2 Recognise my own needs as an individual – that is, separate from what is expected of me in particular roles, such as partner, parent, son or daughter.
3 Make clear 'I' statements about how I feel and what I think, for example 'I feel very uncomfortable with your decision.'
4 Allow myself to make mistakes, recognising that it is normal to make mistakes.
5 Change my mind if I choose to.
6 Ask for 'thinking-it-over time'. For example, when people ask me to do something, I have the right to say 'I would like to think it over and I will let you know by the end of the week.'
7 Allow myself to enjoy my successes – that is, by being pleased with what I have done and sharing it with others.
8 Ask for what I want rather than hoping someone will notice what I want.
9 Recognise that I am not responsible for the behaviour of other adults.
10 Respect other people and their right to be assertive and expect the same in return.
11 Say I don't understand.
12 Deal with others without being dependent on them for approval.

Currently, how much do you believe each of these rules and put them into practice?

I have the right to:	Do I believe this rule is true?		Have I applied this in the last week?	
1 Respect myself	Yes ☐	No ☐	Yes ☐	No ☐
2 Recognise my own needs as an individual independent of others	Yes ☐	No ☐	Yes ☐	No ☐
3 Make clear 'I' statements about how I feel and what I think, for example 'I feel very uncomfortable with your decision'	Yes ☐	No ☐	Yes ☐	No ☐
4 Allow myself to make mistakes	Yes ☐	No ☐	Yes ☐	No ☐
5 Change my mind	Yes ☐	No ☐	Yes ☐	No ☐
6 Ask for 'thinking-it-over time'	Yes ☐	No ☐	Yes ☐	No ☐
7 Allow myself to enjoy my successes	Yes ☐	No ☐	Yes ☐	No ☐
8 Ask for what I want, rather than hoping someone will notice what I want	Yes ☐	No ☐	Yes ☐	No ☐
9 Recognise that I am not responsible for the behaviour of other adults	Yes ☐	No ☐	Yes ☐	No ☐
10 Respect other people and their right to be assertive and expect the same in return	Yes ☐	No ☐	Yes ☐	No ☐
11 Say I don't understand	Yes ☐	No ☐	Yes ☐	No ☐
12 Deal with others without being dependent on them for approval	Yes ☐	No ☐	Yes ☐	No ☐

It is possible to put these rights into practice by using a number of assertiveness techniques.

EXPERIMENT

It may be that you have fears of how others may see or react to you if you become more assertive. The best way of challenging these fears is to note them but act against them by being assertive. Experiment and test out what happens. You may be surprised!

The following are some techniques you can use to develop your assertiveness skills:

Starting and maintaining conversations

Sometimes we can feel isolated, with no one around to talk to. We may have felt lonely for a long time and have a lack of contact with others. There are all sorts of practical things you can do to begin to meet people.

Suggestions might include the following:

- Make new friends through people you know already.
- Join clubs or sign up for further education college courses.
- Look out for local places where you can meet others, e.g. community organisations or your local place of worship. Some local businesses, such as pharmacies and hairdressers, also provide a place to talk.
- Re-establish contact with people you know from your past. Use email, letters or the telephone. Arrange to meet if possible.

The workbook *Practical problem-solving* will help you plan to do this. However, sometimes doing all this can be easier said (or written) than done. We often know we need to go out, join a group or take up an interest, but often we do not know what to do in order to start a meaningful conversation when we get there.

Think about some good conversation starters – 'How are you?', 'Nice day, isn't it?', 'Hi! I'm new here and a little bit nervous'. Remember – it doesn't matter if you talk about superficial things like the weather or football to begin with.

If this is an issue for you, consider planning some **conversation starters in advance**. Good opening questions often begin with the words:

- **What** (e.g. 'What was the meeting like last week?', 'What did you think of that sermon?', 'What did you do yesterday?').
- **How** (e.g. 'How did you find the concert?', 'How are you?', 'How was the talk?').
- **When** (e.g. 'When are you away next?', 'When will we be covering Abba's music on the course?').
- **Who** (e.g. 'Who came yesterday?', 'Who is that over there?').
- **Why** (e.g. 'Why does that happen?', 'Why do we do things this way?', 'Why did Abba split up at the height of their powers?').

These can be followed by **backup questions**, e.g. 'Who came yesterday?', 'Did they enjoy it?', 'What did they say?', 'Did it go well?', 'Do you think they'll come back?'

Sometimes, making these changes can seem very scary and off-putting. If so, you need to think about making changes in a step-by-step way that slowly builds your confidence. The workbook *Overcoming reduced activity and avoidance* will help you with ideas of how to do this.

Assertiveness techniques you can plan to use

Once you get into conversation, the following assertive techniques will help you to build assertive communication into what you say.

Broken record

This is a useful technique and can work in virtually any situation. You practise what it is you want to say by repeating over and over again what it is you want or need. During the conversation, keep returning to your prepared lines, stating clearly and precisely exactly what it is you need or want. Do not be put off by clever arguments or by what the other person says. Once you have prepared the lines you want to say, you can relax. There is nothing that can defeat this tactic!

 EXAMPLE

Anne: 'Can I borrow £10 from you?'

Paul: 'I cannot lend you any money: I've run out.'

Anne: 'I'll pay you back as soon as I can. I need it desperately. You are my friend, aren't you?'

Paul: 'I cannot lend you any money.'

Anne: 'I would do the same for you. You won't miss £10.'

Paul: 'I am your friend, but I cannot lend you any money. I'm afraid I've run out . . . and I've lost my wallet again!'

Remember:
- Work out beforehand what you want to say.
- Repeat your reply over and over again, and stick to what you have decided.

This approach is particularly useful in:
- Situations where your rights are being ignored.
- Coping with clever people who can out-argue you.

Scripting

Scripting involves planning out in advance, in your mind or on paper, exactly what you want to say. This four-stage plan covers:
- **The event:** the situation, relationship or practical problem that is important to you.
- **Your feelings:** how you feel about a situation or problem.
- **Your needs:** what you want to happen in order to make things different.
- **The consequences:** how making these positive changes will improve the situation for you and/or for others.
- **The event:** say what it is you are talking about. Let the other person know precisely what situation you are referring to.
- **Your feelings:** express how the event mentioned affects your own feelings. Opinions can be argued with, but feelings cannot. Expressing your feelings clearly can prevent a lot of confusion.
- **Your needs:** people aren't mind-readers. You need to tell them what you need, otherwise this can lead to resentment and misunderstanding.
- **The consequences:** tell the person that there will be a positive consequence for both of you. Be clear about the consequences.

A good way to begin to practise scripting is to **write down** what you want to say **before** you go into a situation.

 EXAMPLE

Anne: 'Hello. How are you?'

Joan: 'All right. And you?'

Anne: 'I saw Sandra yesterday. She said she was sorry to hear that I wasn't getting on with my neighbour. I told you about that in confidence. I didn't expect you to go round telling others.' **[Event]**

Joan: 'I thought Sandra was a good friend of yours. I didn't think you would mind. She asked how you were and said you seemed troubled. It seemed natural to tell her. Why?'

Anne: 'Sandra's OK but she has a tendency to discuss other people's problems with everyone she meets. I feel angry and upset that you have discussed this with her and let down by you as a friend.' **[Feeling]**

Joan: 'I didn't realise. I'm sorry.'

Anne: 'I value our friendship and the fact that usually I can talk to you about things without you telling everyone else about it.'

Joan: 'Yes, and I feel the same. I don't know what made me say anything to Sandra. She seemed genuinely concerned.'

Anne: 'I'd like us to remain friends and to be able to share problems, but I need to feel I can trust you.' **[Need]**

Joan: 'I won't make this mistake again. Let's not spoil our friendship over this.'

Anne: 'We can stay friends, but I would appreciate it if you didn't discuss my problems with others. Then we can both benefit from a friendship where we know a confidence will not be betrayed.' **[Consequence]**

 Before you move on, write out an **assertive script** using the headings 'event', 'feelings', 'needs' and 'consequences'. Sometimes things can look good on paper but not really flow naturally when you speak them out loud. To test this, speak out loud to yourself and see how your script flows. You might consider acting it out with a friend and having them respond in various different ways – from complete agreement through to disagreement. This will allow you to plan how to respond. If you can practise this with a friend, ask them to comment on how you come over (e.g. too loud or too fast). Also, ask them about any non-verbal aspects you should change (e.g. eye contact; see below).

Saying no

Many people find that 'no' seems to be one of the hardest words to say. We can sometimes be drawn into situations that we don't want to be in because we avoid saying this one simple word. The images we associate with saying no may prevent us from using the word when we need it. We may be scared of being seen as mean and selfish or of being rejected by others. Saying no can be both important and helpful.

 Do I have problems saying no?   Yes ☐   No ☐   Sometimes ☐

If you do, try to practise saying no by using the following principles:

- Be straightforward and honest so that you can make your point effectively. That isn't the same as being rude.
- Tell the person if you are finding it difficult.
- Don't apologise and give all sorts of reasons for saying no. It is OK to say no if you don't want to do things.
- Remember that it is better in the long run to be truthful than to breed resentment and bitterness within yourself.

Body language and assertiveness

How we communicate involves more than just words. Our tone of voice, the speed and volume at which we speak, our eye contact and our body posture all contribute to how we come over. When you are being assertive, be aware of the non-verbal communications you make as well as the words you say.

- **Eye contact:** meet the other person's eyes from time to time. Make eye contact, but don't end up staring at the person. Try not to look down for long, as this may communicate weakness to others. If you find this difficult, practise looking just past the person. For example, look at an object such as a picture on the wall behind them.
- **Your voice:** try to vary your tone so you come over well. Don't be afraid of silence – especially if you have asked a question. You need to be aware in advance of the strange change that

happens to the physics of time when we feel anxious. If we ask a question, we may find ourselves tempted to fill uncomfortable gaps. Even two seconds can feel too long. Knowing this helps you to be prepared to allow a little silence. Likewise, you don't need to reply instantly to any question asked of you. You're allowed some time to think. Other aspects of your voice also matter. Consider how quickly and loudly you talk. Anxiety or anger may cause you to speed up and gabble your words or to slow down so you come over as hesitant. Either extreme will affect how you come over. Aim for a relaxed and yet serious manner if you can.

- **Posture:** think about how you hold your body. Try to look up and don't hunch over, which can occur when we feel vulnerable or anxious. Keep an appropriate distance (personal space) between you and the other person. Don't get too close, as this might be seen as aggressive or inappropriate (unless you know the person very well).
- **Be friendly:** smile once in a while.
- **Be relaxed in your body:** have a relaxed body posture. Think about how you hold your body. Clenched fists and a frown may be caused by tension and anxiety but may come over as aggression. Relax your body. Quickly screen how you are holding your arms and shoulders and try to relax tense muscles. If it's an important meeting, consider using a relaxation tape beforehand to relax your body as well as your mind.

 IMPORTANT POINT

It can be easy for our non-verbal messages to either reinforce or cancel out the messages we are trying to convey. However, don't think you have to get all this right straight away. You can slowly make these changes over a number of weeks or even months. You don't want to get confused because you are concerned about whether you are avoiding eye contact enough! All you need to do is be aware of this as an issue and try occasionally to make some small changes in what you do. Experiment and see what works for you.

Putting into practice what you have learned

You have now covered the key elements of assertiveness. In planning to be assertive, there are a few other things to bear in mind. This involves considering the following when you plan to respond assertively.

Choose:

- **The right person:** we all know that some people can take even assertive feedback badly. If you know that what you say is likely to be misinterpreted or that they will overreact, then you need to recruit some extra help such as a close friend or another family member.
- **The right time:** for example, don't raise important issues immediately after your partner returns from work or the pub. Choose a more relaxed time or engineer such a time – for example, go for a walk together.
- **The right issue:** the issue needs to be something that the other person can change. For example, asking them to lose three stone and stop smoking immediately is not realistic. Instead, discuss your concerns for their health and say how you are prepared to help them change to cut down smoking if they want to.
- **The right words:** use the approaches described in this workbook (broken record, scripting and saying no). These techniques will give you the tools to say what you need.

Think about how you can be more assertive in your own life. If you recognise that a lack of assertiveness is a problem for you, try to:

- Use one of the assertiveness techniques during the next week.

● Remind yourself about and put into practice the **rules of assertion**. Copy or tear out page 5 and carry it around with you. Put it somewhere where you will see it, such as by the television, on a door or mirror, or on the fridge, to remind you of the rules.

 Credit-card-sized versions of the rules of assertion and the seven steps of problem-solving are available for you to print off free of charge or order from www.livinglifetothefull.com.

After you have tried this approach for a week, read the next section of the workbook to review your progress.

Section 2 My review of my assertive practice

In the first part of this workbook, you learned that assertiveness is being able to stand up for yourself by making sure your opinions and feelings are considered. Assertion is not about winning, but it is concerned with being able to walk away feeling that you have put across what you wanted to say.

Review of the rules of assertion

The following table contains the **rules of assertion**. Look through them and then tick those rules that you have, or could have, put into practice over the last week.

I have the right to:	Do I believe this rule is true?		Have I applied this in the last week?	
1 Respect myself	Yes ☐	No ☐	Yes ☐	No ☐
2 Recognise my own needs as an individual independent of others	Yes ☐	No ☐	Yes ☐	No ☐
3 Make clear 'I' statements about how I feel and what I think, for example 'I feel very uncomfortable with your decision'	Yes ☐	No ☐	Yes ☐	No ☐
4 Allow myself to make mistakes	Yes ☐	No ☐	Yes ☐	No ☐
5 Change my mind	Yes ☐	No ☐	Yes ☐	No ☐
6 Ask for thinking-it-over time	Yes ☐	No ☐	Yes ☐	No ☐
7 Allow myself to enjoy my successes	Yes ☐	No ☐	Yes ☐	No ☐
8 Ask for what I want, rather than hoping someone will notice what I want	Yes ☐	No ☐	Yes ☐	No ☐
9 Recognise that I am not responsible for the behaviour of other adults	Yes ☐	No ☐	Yes ☐	No ☐
10 Respect other people and their right to be assertive and expect the same in return	Yes ☐	No ☐	Yes ☐	No ☐
11 Say I don't understand	Yes ☐	No ☐	Yes ☐	No ☐
12 Deal with others without being dependent on them for approval	Yes ☐	No ☐	Yes ☐	No ☐

If you could have been more assertive this week but avoided putting the rules of assertion into practice, this shows that you need to continue to work on this area.

(**?**) Were you able to act in an assertive way at some stage in the past week?   Yes ☐   No ☐

(?) If yes, were you able to respond:

	Yes ☐	No ☐	Sometimes ☐
Directly and openly?	Yes ☐	No ☐	Sometimes ☐
Respecting your own opinions and rights and expecting others to do the same?	Yes ☐	No ☐	Sometimes ☐

(?) What was the impact on you?

✎

....

....

....

(?) What was the impact on others?

✎

....

....

....

(?) Did you fear that if you were assertive, it would go badly wrong?　　　　Yes ☐　　No ☐　　Sometimes ☐

(?) If yes, was this fear accurate and/or helpful?　　　Accurate ☐　Inaccurate ☐ or
　　　　　　　　　　　　　　　　　　　Helpful ☐　　Unhelpful ☐

Often, one of the reasons why a person avoids being assertive is that they **fear** the consequences. They may mind-read that others will dislike them or reject them, or they may have catastrophic fears about the consequences of assertion. As with most fears, they are both extreme and unhelpful. One problem is that unless the person is able to identify and question their fearful thoughts, they may **avoid** being assertive as a consequence. The very best way to challenge these thoughts is to **undermine** them by **choosing** to be assertive and discovering what happens.

Workbook summary

In this workbook, you have:
- Discovered the differences between passive, aggressive, passive-aggressive and assertive styles of behaviour.
- Learned the rules of assertion and how you can put them into practice in everyday situations.
- Practised assertive techniques in your own life.
- Reviewed your own style of communicating with others.

Putting into practice what you have learned

Re-read what you learned earlier in the workbook about the **broken record** and **scripting** approaches and try to put them into practice during the next week. In particular, the scripting approach allows you to plan out how to be assertive in a particular situation and with a specific person. View this as a sort of action plan that can help both of you to change how you are and also to learn something new about yourself and other people.

If relationships are a problem for you, consider reading the *Building relationships* workbook with your partner. Read it through together. You might also want to go through the workbook *Information for families and friends – how can I offer support?*.

Acknowledgements

I wish to thank all those who have commented upon this workbook, especially Marie Chellingsworth, Jeanette Wallis and Dr Nicky Dummett.

My notes

....
....
....
....
....
....
....
....
....
....
....
....
....
....
....
....
....
....
....
....
....
....
....
....
....
....
....
....
....
....

My notes

....

Building relationships

Dr Chris Williams

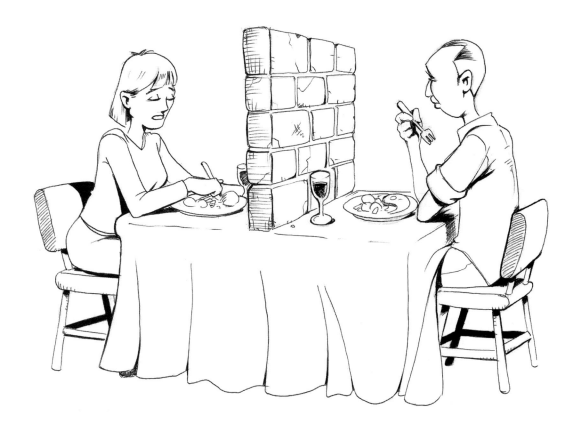

A Five Areas Approach
Helping you to help yourself
www.livinglifetothefull.com

Section *1*   **Introduction**

We are usually happiest in life when our relationships with others feel 'right'. Remember the happiness and excitement that we feel when a relationship starts? And the upset when a relationship ends, and the stress when things are going wrong? Many readers may find they are in such a situation. This workbook is written for you.

In this workbook you will:

- Discover your relationship style – which affects how you relate to others.
- Find out how past relationships affect our current relationships.
- Learn how to build (and rebuild) relationships by building communication and commitment.

Our relationship styles

We are all different. Some of us have many friends and acquaintances. Others prefer to keep to ourselves and have fewer people around who are 'close'. Whatever sort of style of relationship you prefer, it can be affected during times of upset.

Our past and present relationships are some of the most powerful factors that affect how we feel. Our early relationships influence how we relate to others in other ways too. They teach us styles of relating that cause us to repeat patterns in how we relate to others.

Our upbringing teaches us rules about:

- How we should communicate with others – with assertiveness, passivity or aggression (see the workbook *Being assertive*).
- How we expect others to relate to us – whether they are trustworthy or will let us down.

These rules may include helpful and positive rules, for example that we are loved, trusted and accepted. However, sometimes the rules we learn are more negative and unhelpful.

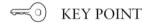 KEY POINT

Most of us learn a mixture of both helpful and unhelpful rules. These can affect how we react to others, especially when we are upset.

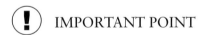 IMPORTANT POINT

Use the checklist below to identify your own helpful and unhelpful styles of relating.

What we have learnt from past experience	How this affects our relationships now (our relationship style)	Tick here if this applies to you – even if only sometimes
We may learn generally positive things about how we see ourselves, others and relationships. We have a reasonable self-esteem.	We generally like ourselves and have a good self-esteem. We think generally positively of others while realising that we and they have faults. We are able to trust others and make a commitment in relationships. This is a healthy state to be in and to aim for.	

What we have learnt from past experience	How this affects our relationships now (our relationship style)	Tick here if this applies to you – even if only sometimes
We may develop a low sense of worth/self-esteem. For example, we may doubt whether we can be loved. We may believe we are unattractive, boring or unlovable. There may be all sorts of fears that if others knew the 'real' us they would run a mile.	The result is that we put on a front and cannot be ourselves. We end up being clingy and dependent in relationships and passively do anything to keep a partner happy. We may use alcohol or drugs because we think they make us more interesting.	
We develop the opposite of this – a high but fragile self-esteem that is linked to an inner neediness. We may have been taught as a child that we can do anything and the whole world revolves around us. We see ourselves as special. If there are difficulties, they are caused by others.	We can be very demanding of others. Things must revolve around us. We need to get our own way. We are often impatient with others who don't see the point. We may seek out passive partners who will look up to us and do what we want. At the same time, we may know we could always do better. Job titles and roles really matter, and yet we may quickly feel dissatisfied with jobs and people and want to move on.	
We think of ourselves as ugly, unattractive or unlovable.	We may feel uncomfortable with and avoid close relationships and commitment to protect ourselves from hurt ('It will never last'). We are uncomfortable being touched intimately by others. We may dress down and cover up any attractive features by wearing looser clothes. We may give up and let ourselves go. Alternatively, we may become obsessed that we must look just right. We may flirt or sleep around to test out whether we are really attractive or constantly test the love of those who care for us.	
Sometimes events in our own lives may have taught us rules that others are untrustworthy. We may have learned that people we love let us down or abandon us.	The result is that we may well find it difficult to commit or respond with trust to others, even when they want to make a commitment to us. Our lack of trust may end up driving them away.	
Sometimes our doubts can lead to jealous worries or anger.	Jealousy comes from fear and can severely damage our relationships. We may make demands that our partner never goes out alone, especially with people of the opposite sex. We may accuse our partner of being attracted to others or become obsessed with pampering and pleasing them in clingy ways that suffocate and restrict.	

What we have learnt from past experience	How this affects our relationships now (our relationship style)	Tick here if this applies to you – even if only sometimes
The past may have taught us that others use us sexually. We may have learned that sex is something to just do or have done to us. We may have been taught that sex is dirty or wrong or that it is about power, winning and getting your own way.	The result may be to withdraw from the possibility of sex. We cannot enjoy this aspect of our lives. These rules may prevent us from developing a sex life where we can have trust, commitment and enjoyment. Sometimes we end up in patterns of relationships with partners who make demands and do not respect us.	
'I must not show my emotions': we may have learned it is dangerous to expose our emotions or that being seen to be upset is a sign of weakness.	The stereotype is that men bottle up their emotions and use alcohol or work to block out how they feel, whereas women are happier discussing their emotions and relationships with others. Of course, both patterns can occur with either gender. What matters more is the match (or **mismatch**) between two people. For example, when one partner feels distressed and is struggling to cope, they may desperately want to discuss issues in their relationship, life, etc., but their partner may not want or feel able to. This clash of styles can lead to further difficulties.	

 LEARNING POINT

Repeating patterns in relationships

These rules can explain why sometimes we repeat the same patterns in relationships over and over. They can help us understand why we always go for the same type of person and why sometimes we keep making the same mistakes. Being aware of these patterns is the first step towards changing them. We can learn new rules.

It is important to be aware of the rules and beliefs you have about you, your family, friends and relatives. They will affect the styles and patterns of relating you have in relationships.

How do I relate to others I am emotionally close to?

The following questions will help you to consider your own attitudes and reactions towards others you are close to, for example a partner, son, daughter or parent. It may be tempting to answer these questions quite quickly with what you perceive to be the 'correct' answer. You'll get the most from this, though, if you really reflect on the questions. The purpose isn't to make you feel bad about yourself but instead to help you to begin to think about things that may need to change in order for you to build more balanced relationships.

How do I respond to people I get close to? And how do they respond to me?

Think back on your current and past close relationships.

(?) What **helpful** relationship styles do you repeat?

✎

....

....

....

(?) What **unhelpful** relationship styles do you repeat?

✎

....

....

....

(?) How do these patterns affect your relationships, both now and in the past?

✎

....

....

....

(?) How might these factors affect how you respond when you feel distressed?

✎

....

....

....

(?) Do you regularly feel uncomfortable when speaking about how you or they feel?

✎

....

....

....

(?) Do you try to avoid speaking about how you feel? How do those around you react to this?

....

....

....

☞ KEY POINT

These unhelpful patterns may not affect us for much of the time. However, they can come to the surface when we feel more distressed. When this happens, they can unhelpfully disrupt how we react to those who we are close to.

What factors have shaped my attitudes and responses?

Think about the things from the past (e.g. upbringing, childhood memories, comments that parents have made) that may affect how you approach close relationships.

(?) How has my own upbringing affected my own view of how to relate to those I am close to?

....

....

....

Things you can do that can make a difference

The following are some things you can do (and not do) in order to build relationships.

With people you don't know so well

Do:

- Be yourself.
- Have planned a brief one-line statement of how you are if someone asks 'How are you?' Remember: they don't know you well. They may well not be aware that you are finding things difficult at the moment. Don't feel you have to tell the person everything about yourself. Say something like 'Getting on fine, thanks. How are you? Great weather isn't it?', and leave it at that.

Don't:

- Tell everyone about every aspect of your life and how you feel – they're only the milkman, not your therapist!

With trusted friends and family members

Our wider family and friends can be a great support for us. A workbook *Information for families and friends – how can I offer support?* has been written for them. You might wish to show that workbook to them or even plan to go through it together.

Do:
- Find support from close friends.

Don't:
- Become dependent on others or think that only they can help.
- Become overly focused on just one friendship.
- Mix up friendship and sex. The last thing you need is the complexity of finding that a good confiding friendship has been altered forever by something that has 'just happened'.

With partners

Our partners are often our closest supports and companions. Because of this, the relationship can have a large impact on how each of us feels. Sometimes, these closest relationships develop problems. These include anger, jealousy, boredom, breakups and affairs. These problems are often the result of a breakdown of communication and even love.

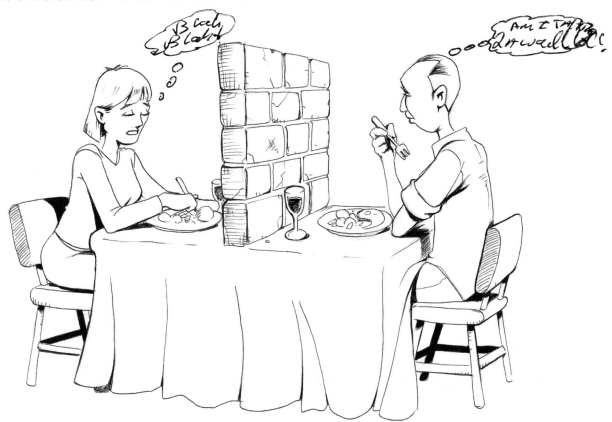

- **Poor communication:** this can happen in any relationship, but it becomes even more pronounced when we are low or stressed. We may not feel like talking, or we lack the energy or motivation to talk for long. Sometimes these changes happen suddenly. More often, however, they build up slowly over months and years. You may find you have nothing to say or even that you do not know how to start a conversation with your partner. Your partner feels like a stranger.
- **Sex:** you may lose interest in sex or become anxious about your ability to perform. Sometimes, medications can cause impotence or prevent orgasm. It may become tempting to spice up a relationship with flirtation or pornography. Online porn and chat rooms may provide a sense of emotional closeness with someone you have never met. You may be tempted to use telephone sex lines or dating agencies promising 'discreet' relationships. Sometimes people try to jolt themselves out of low mood by having a one-night stand or starting an affair. Your partner may have reacted similarly and you may have discovered they have had an affair.

- **Time apart:** A symptom of a relationship in trouble is making choices not to be around each other as much. We may work late or go out more. Sometimes people cope by throwing themselves into looking after their children. Children may provide the sense of emotional connection that is missing in their relationship. People can drift apart even when they are in the same room, for example they may never talk while watching television.

Ultimately, these issues come down to issues of **communication** and **commitment**.

Rebuilding relationships by building communication and commitment

A key question is how much improvement you both feel you need to make in order to improve things. To rebuild (or build) a relationship can sometimes come down to one partner making changes by themselves. However, that really misses the point of the need for both partners to discuss and work on these issues together.

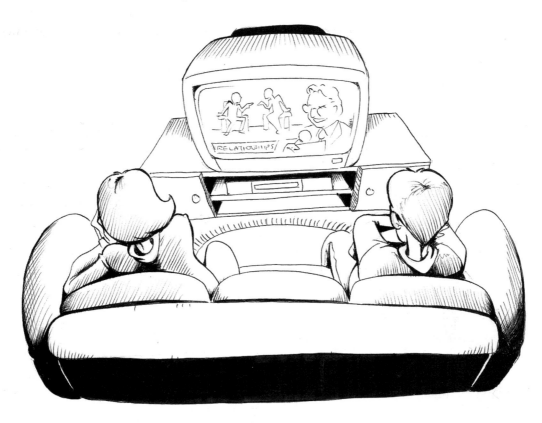

It may be that only some small changes of direction are needed. If so, some immediate things you can do with your partner include:

- Listening: pay attention – don't just switch off and think you know what is being said. Talk about each other's days. Ask questions about the small but important details in life.
- Doing things together: **spend time together going for walks or eating meals together.**
- **Tackling 'relationship killers',** such as doing things apart.
- Forgiving: living with anger and guilt can eat away at a relationship. You may need to forgive your partner or ask for forgiveness from them if you have done things that have caused hurt.
- Developing physical intimacy in your everyday life at a level that you both feel happy with. Hugs, kisses and holding hands can help build bridges. If you have lost your sex drive because of how you feel, try to discuss this. Be clear that it isn't that you don't find your partner attractive or care for them. Try to agree that although you may not have sex very often (or even at all), you can still hug and kiss. Even if you lack interest in sex, your partner has sexual needs too: try finding substitutes for full intercourse that satisfy their sexual needs.

● Bringing the romance back into what you do: add surprises, meals out, weekends away, compliments, a nicely cooked meal or occasional small gifts. It's the thought and preparation time that matter here, not the cost. Extravagant gifts are no replacement for time together.

Hearing what we expect to hear

At the heart of many relationship difficulties is a lack of communication. When people have drifted apart, there is likely to be blame on both sides, and people may feel hurt. When someone is distressed, they tend to interpret things in extreme and unhelpful ways. This can affect strongly how we interpret even the same conversation. We may think we know each other so well that we assume we know what is going to be said. The trouble is that sometimes we can be wrong. We don't actually listen to what the other person is really saying. For example, one partner may say 'That was a nice meal' and mean it as a compliment. However, because of suspicion, hurt and upset, their partner may hear it as 'Well, you've cooked something nice for once. Usually you don't make much effort.' Sometimes people can be indirectly aggressive and sarcastic when they offer compliments. The danger is that all sorts of positive or neutral replies are interpreted in a negative way.

 EXPERIMENT

Try this test to see whether you and your partner interpret the same event in the same way. Look in depth at a time when you both felt hurt, angry or upset. Do this when the heat has gone out of the episode. First, both of you should separately complete the thought-review worksheet on page 35 of the workbook *Noticing and changing extreme and unhelpful thinking*. When you have done this, compare what you have both written. A copy is also included on the final page of this workbook.

Look at how you both interpreted what happened. How did this affect how you felt and what you did? Do you both agree on what happened? Is there is a difference in how you both see things? Can this help to explain your reactions? Could this difference in perception be happening again and again?

If this is an issue, first identify it as a problem. You can do this by choosing to clarify and check out what you both mean. This will help you to avoid jumping to conclusions about each other. Don't do this in an accusatory way. Instead, agree that if either of you isn't quite sure of what the other really means, then you will ask. Ask politely – not in an angry or defensive way.

Try to restrain any immediate reactions to rise to any perceived hurt or insult. Check it out. If they are trying to be critical, then this will quickly come out, but often you may find that miscommunication is rife.

Some difficult issues

● If your partner feels like a stranger to you and you want to rebuild things, you both need to go back to the basics. Be open and discuss how you feel. Decide jointly what you want to do about things. If you both want to tackle this, then agree some ground rules. These rules should cover time together, sharing household tasks and childcare responsibilities, eating together and issues such as sex. Slowly, it is possible to rebuild a sense of love. Expect things to be difficult for some time as you both try to make the changes needed.

● There may have been an affair or one of you may have moved out. There may be a lot of emotional hurt. Again, you both need to be open, discuss how you feel, and talk about what you want to do about things. Can things recover? Or is it too late? These are times of great challenge in the relationship for both of you. Sometimes, relationships end at this stage in recrimination and anger – or just a sense of sadness. Sometimes, they can move to friendship. Often, things can still be rebuilt. Time can heal things.

- If there is violence towards you, then you need to be clear that this is unacceptable. **If you are being threatened or hit,** you should seriously consider leaving home or ask your partner to leave, at least for a time. Men can be abused too, and they may feel shame and isolation. Any violence or aggression is unacceptable. If children are involved, you need to make sure that they are protected. Many people feel powerless and stuck in such relationships – or too scared to leave. If you are in this situation, seek professional help. Options include talking to your doctor, social services or the police. If you are scared of contacting these services, talk things through with a trusted friend and ask them to go with you. One thing you can be certain about is that unless things change, your relationship will end up being destroyed one way or another. The telephone directory lists the numbers of local domestic violence helplines and support agencies. These are confidential and can be a good source of advice. The National Domestic Violence Helpline is at 0808 2000 247 or www.womensaid.org.uk.

- **If you are hitting or harming your partner or children,** then you need to recognise that this is unacceptable. This violence may be a new behaviour that is the result of the anger linked to depression or tension. Sometimes it is the result of alcohol. Violence and threats may be something that you have done for a long time and in a variety of relationships. Either way, the key thing is to recognise that you are hurting the people that you love and must stop. Look for times when you are prone to losing control (e.g. after drinking alcohol) and tackle this. Anger-management groups and strategies can help. Please see your doctor about this. Reducing your alcohol intake can help, as can treating any depression or anxiety. You will feel better for it – and you may be able to save and rebuild your relationship too.

Sometimes the extent of the relationship breakdown may be that we need professional advice, such as counselling. Here, charities such as Relate can be helpful. Although many relationships can be rebuilt, sometimes they cannot and a time apart or permanent separation may result.

To find your nearest Relate Centre, call Relate general enquiries on 0845 456 1310 (local rate applies) or look at www.relate.org.uk. For a telephone counselling appointment, call 0845 130 4016.

Workbook summary

In this workbook you have:
- Discovered your relationship style – which affects how you relate to others.
- Found out how past relationships affect our current relationships.
- Learned how to build and rebuild relationships by building communication and commitment.

Putting into practice what you have learned

Some of the changes described in this workbook will seem straightforward and others more difficult. You may feel scared about making these changes. Other workbooks in the course may help, especially *Helpful and unhelpful behaviours* and *Overcoming reduced activity and avoidance*.

You may find that showing this workbook to a trusted friend or relative may help you to work out some ideas for making changes.

Remember to use the blank thought review worksheet at the end of the workbook if there is a possibility that you and someone close to you are misinterpreting things.

Acknowledgements

I wish to thank all who have commented on this workbook, especially Marie Chellingsworth, Dr Nicky Dummett and Jeanette Wallis.

My notes

....
....
....
....
....
....
....
....
....
....
....
....
....
....
....
....
....
....
....
....
....
....
....
....
....
....
....
....
....
....

A specific time when I and someone I am close to have responded with upset.

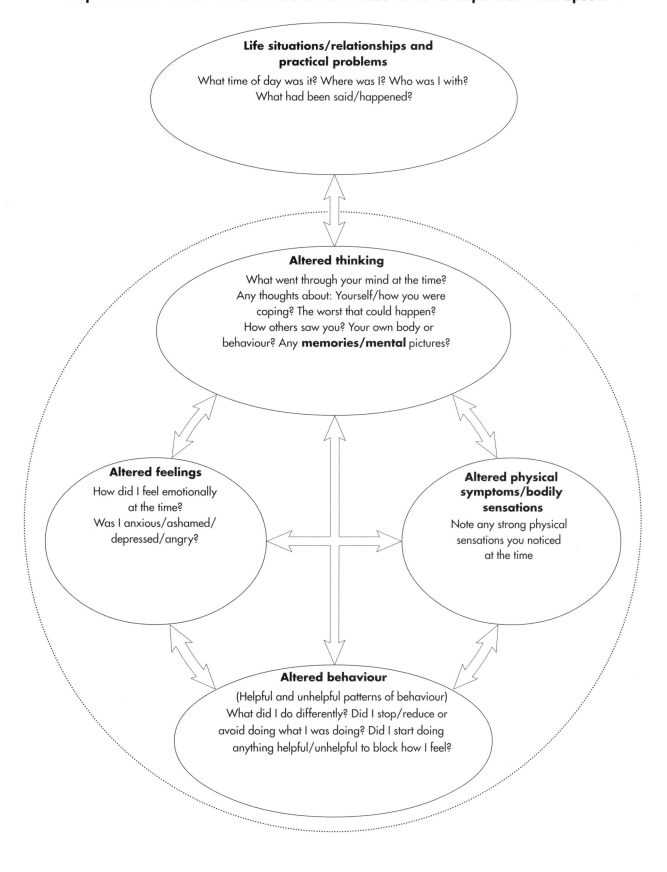

Life situations/relationships and
practical problems

What time of day was it? Where was I? Who was I with?
What had been said/happened?

Altered thinking

What went through your mind at the time?
Any thoughts about: Yourself/how you were
coping? The worst that could happen?
How others saw you? Your own body or
behaviour? Any **memories/mental** pictures?

Altered feelings

How did I feel emotionally
at the time?
Was I anxious/ashamed/
depressed/angry?

Altered physical
symptoms/bodily
sensations

Note any strong physical
sensations you noticed
at the time

Altered behaviour

(Helpful and unhelpful patterns of behaviour)
What did I do differently? Did I stop/reduce or
avoid doing what I was doing? Did I start doing
anything helpful/unhelpful to block how I feel?

Information for families and friends: how can I offer support?

Dr Chris Williams

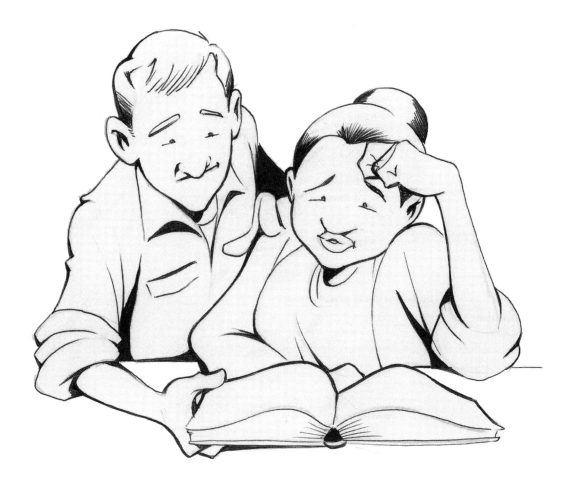

A Five Areas Approach
Helping you to help yourself
www.livinglifetothefull.com

Section *1*   **Introduction**

This workbook is written for the families and friends of people who are feeling unwell. It summarises the key elements of the course approach, so that relatives and friends can understand and offer support in the best possible way.

In this workbook you will learn:

- What this course is about – and how the person is using it.
- How best to help and communicate effectively.
- Helpful and unhelpful things you can do so that you can offer effective support.
- How to look after yourself as a friend or relative so that you stay well.
- How to put into practice what you've learned.

Background for friends and family

The course workbooks use a proven approach based on cognitive behaviour therapy (CBT). This is an effective form of treatment that can be helpful for people who are facing a wide range of difficulties, including physical health problems, stress and low mood. When symptoms have ground down a person for a long time, it can be hard for them to be objective, both about the current situation and about how things were in the past. An important aspect of your role as a supporter is to provide support and an objective viewpoint. This can help encourage the person and keep them on track in working on their difficulties.

The approach used in the course looks in detail at five key areas of our lives. The **five areas assessment** provides a clear summary of the range of difficulties a person may face in each of the following areas:

- Life situation, relationships, practical problems and difficulties.
- Symptoms in the body.
- Altered thinking (with extreme and unhelpful thinking).
- Altered feelings (also called moods or emotions).
- Altered behaviour or activity levels.

What we think about a situation or problem may affect how we feel emotionally and physically. It can also alter what we do.

The five areas assessment model

Because of the links between each of the areas, the actions that we take can worsen or keep our symptoms going. Importantly, it also means that helpful changes in any one of the areas can lead to benefits in the others as well.

About the workbook approach

The course workbooks aim to help people to bring about change in these five key areas. They are practical workbooks, which involve stopping, thinking and reflecting on the impact that symptoms can have. They also teach key changes that can make a difference.

The workbooks are usually used by the person on their own and aim to help them:

● Discover new useful information.
● Develop important new life skills that they can then use to make changes in these different areas of their lives.

Workbooks are used one at a time, and the reader is encouraged to read them slowly. This allows them to put what they have learned into practice over a week or so before moving on. The workbooks can also be discussed (if the person wants) with other people, such as family members, friends and healthcare practitioners. The workbook is the person's own resource and is private to them. Some people find it helpful to share their workbooks; however, you need to respect their wishes here. In the same way as we would never dream of reading someone's personal diary, we should have a similar view when it comes to their workbooks.

In contrast, this current workbook is designed to be read and discussed jointly.

Section 2 How we can help

All of us are surrounded by people and have all sorts of different friendships and relationships. The most important relationships are often with those people we either live with or have a lot of contact with, especially our friends, family members and partners. When someone we know develops symptoms, it can be difficult to know how best to help. Their problems can affect us too.

A common difficulty when someone is struggling is that their family or friends may not understand fully what is happening or know how to offer help. We may have never experienced ourselves what the person is going through. This can lead to further problems, such as frustration and withdrawal. Sometimes the person who is unwell can become preoccupied with how they feel and struggle to communicate. Seeing each other's points of view at times like this is important. The danger is when either party starts to think that those around them no longer care. Stating clearly what we are thinking and feeling here can be really important. If you are someone who thinks that you are not able to talk through how things are – or you are unsure how either of you can show that you care – then this workbook is for you.

There may be all sorts of other worries. We may be concerned about other people's reactions, for example neighbours, colleagues, bosses, healthcare practitioners, people at your place of worship, and other friends and relatives.

Ideally, we all want to be able to count on others to support us when we are ill. Sometimes, however, we just don't know how best to help. Friends and relatives often (but not always) offer support when someone becomes ill. For example, if someone has flu, others may help by cooking meals, helping with childcare and doing some housework. If an illness lasts for a number of weeks, months or years, then we may find that this practical help is difficult to keep up. Sometimes we may not know how to respond or offer support beyond short-term flowers and get-well cards. Even when we try to help, we may be uncertain how best to do this. We may struggle to know what to say. If you feel like this, you may be tempted to avoid talking about the symptoms and may even avoid visiting the person as a result.

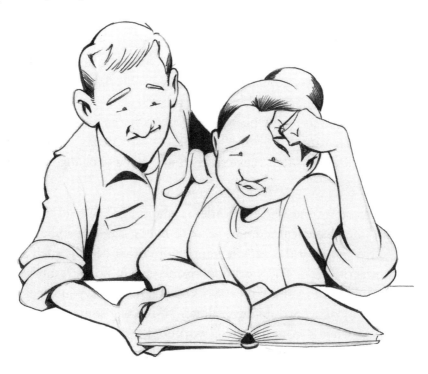

Why emotions are an important part of illness

The five areas diagram on page 3 shows that when we are unwell, there is usually a mix of physical, emotional, behaviour and social impacts.

So, for example, if we have a health problem such as arthritis, heart disease or cancer, we may:

- Notice physical symptoms due to the illness.
- Worry about the future and have all sorts of doubts and fears.
- Alter what we do, by withdrawing from going out, reducing our activity levels or avoiding doing things that seem scary.
- Struggle to cope with feelings of frustration, irritability, anger, shame or upset as we try to come to terms with how we feel.

Similarly, when the main problem is a mental health one such as anxiety or low mood, we may:

- Notice physical symptoms due to the illness, such as poor appetite, weight loss, and problems of physical tension, tiredness or pain.
- Worry about the future and have all sorts of doubts and fears.
- Alter what we do, by withdrawing from going out, reducing our activity levels or avoiding doing things that seem scary.
- Struggle to cope with feelings of frustration, irritability, anger, shame or upset as we try to come to terms with how we feel.

These responses are remarkably similar. Whatever the problems we face, we all need support and understanding from those around us.

Where the illness isn't obvious or believed

When a person has a broken leg, there is a large plaster cast on the leg. With a chest infection, we have lots of green phlegm. In cancer or heart disease, there are cells that are growing too quickly or blocked arteries that cause angina. Sometimes, we have physical illnesses, such as these, that are very visible or can be picked up on scans of the body. However, some symptoms are not so visible, for example problems of tiredness, weakness, dizziness and pain. The same is true of feelings of sadness, stress and tension, which are not visible in the same way as a broken leg, heart disease or cancer.

Because the symptoms are less obvious, sometimes the reaction of others may be less supportive. Sometimes the problem is simply that others just do not know much about these sorts of symptom. Part of this reflects difficulties others may have in understanding how the person feels. The main point is that these problems are just as real as the broken leg or the cancer.

It can be helpful to complete the following checklist together and discuss what you find. Use it as a method of identifying strength areas and possible problems that you may wish to tackle together. If you prefer, you might find it especially helpful to complete the checklist separately and then to discuss together your different answers to each question.

Isolation: the sufferer finds it difficult to really talk and receive support from others	Yes ☐	No ☐	Sometimes ☐
There is just no one around who they can really talk to	Yes ☐	No ☐	Sometimes ☐
Others are unsure how best to offer support	Yes ☐	No ☐	Sometimes ☐
Others have started to drop away from offering support	Yes ☐	No ☐	Sometimes ☐
Others are avoiding talking about the symptoms and their impact	Yes ☐	No ☐	Sometimes ☐
Perhaps even their healthcare practitioners are struggling to offer the kind of support needed	Yes ☐	No ☐	Sometimes ☐
Are their symptoms not visible or obvious to others?	Yes ☐	No ☐	Sometimes ☐
If yes, does this seem to affect how others react?	Yes ☐	No ☐	Sometimes ☐

Write in what you have both noticed here:

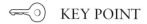

....

....

....

The vicious circle of avoidance

When we feel anxious or worried about things, it is understandable that we tend to avoid situations, people, places or even conversations that we feel may be difficult or stressful. This avoidance adds to our problems because although we may feel less anxious or unwell in the shorter term, in the longer term such actions can worsen the problem. This pattern can lead to a **vicious circle of avoidance**.

KEY POINT

The problem with avoidance is that it teaches you that the only way of dealing with a difficult situation is through avoiding it. Avoidance reduces our opportunities to find out that our worst fears do not occur. Avoidance therefore worsens anxiety and strongly undermines confidence.

EXAMPLE

Mary's and Anne's vicious circles of avoidance

Anne has been struggling to cope with symptoms for several years. She has arthritis, which has made it difficult for her to get out, and she has struggled to keep up with things in her flat. Her sister Mary lives on the other side of town and likes to pop by once every week or so. They have previously got on well, but over recent months Anne has felt increasingly low in mood. Her confidence has taken a huge knock, and she is finding she can no longer cope with things. She tends to sit indoors, crying from time to time. Her symptoms feel far worse, and now she also feels she cannot enjoy things and is struggling to cope. A key issue for Anne is that she feels very embarrassed when things aren't clean and neat in her flat and when she isn't dressed nicely. Now whenever Mary calls by, Anne feels uneasy that she will notice that she isn't coping. She feels deeply ashamed of how things are and is very upset.

Mary is concerned about Anne. She knows that Anne isn't herself. They used to go out together from time to time and really enjoy things. Now the spark seems to have gone out of Anne, and she seems ground down by her symptoms. Mary knows that Anne was badly affected when their brother and his family moved away to the capital earlier in the year. She wants to speak to Anne about how worried she is and how she wants to help. As a family, they have always struggled to be open about how they feel. Although they know they love each other, this isn't something that would usually be said, except perhaps written in birthday and Christmas cards. Now whenever Mary visits Anne, she sits thinking 'We should be discussing things. How can I help?' Mary has tried to bring up her concerns once or twice, but Anne quickly becomes defensive and seems embarrassed.

Both Anne and Mary think 'What can we do?'

Look at the two vicious circles of avoidance that Anne and Mary show.

? How are Anne and Mary's reactions worsening the situation?

✎

....

....

....

? What could they do to change things?

✎

....

....

....

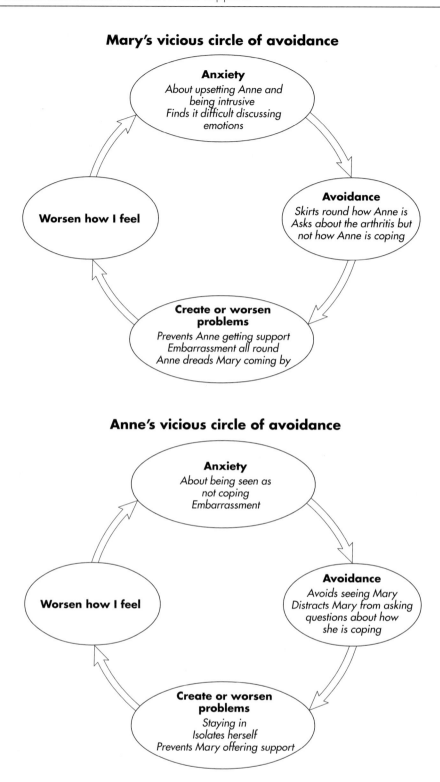

Mary's vicious circle of avoidance

Anxiety
*About upsetting Anne and being intrusive
Finds it difficult discussing emotions*

Avoidance
*Skirts round how Anne is
Asks about the arthritis but not how Anne is coping*

Create or worsen problems
*Prevents Anne getting support
Embarrassment all round
Anne dreads Mary coming by*

Worsen how I feel

Anne's vicious circle of avoidance

Anxiety
*About being seen as not coping
Embarrassment*

Avoidance
*Avoids seeing Mary
Distracts Mary from asking questions about how she is coping*

Create or worsen problems
*Staying in
Isolates herself
Prevents Mary offering support*

Worsen how I feel

Sometimes, even just **talking about the symptoms** can become a topic that is avoided at home or with friends. This can backfire because others may not know or understand the condition we are facing. They may misunderstand, in which case their imaginations may go into overdrive. Misinformation and rumour can create gossip at work or among your neighbours. Even among close relatives and friends there may be embarrassment about discussing things. This is especially the case if our family or personal 'rules' – like Anne's and Mary's – have been to keep the discussion of emotional issues at the level of bunches of flowers and get-well cards. Such gifts are really important, and we can offer only what we can, but sometimes there are also opportunities to change things so that we can offer and receive more helpful support. This may well make us feel anxious, but by making changes slowly one step at a time things can change.

The checklist below describes common areas of avoidance among families and friends. If avoidance is a problem, it is likely that there will be examples of avoidance in at least some of these areas.

As a friend/family member, am I:	Tick here if you have noticed this, even if only sometimes
Completely avoiding asking the sufferer about anything to do with how they feel?	
Avoiding talking to anyone else about the sufferer's symptoms or about how they are coping?	
Putting off all decisions until the person is better, e.g. putting holidays or other life plans completely on hold?	
Not really being honest with others or with the person with symptoms, for example saying yes when really I mean no?	
Trying hard to avoid situations that bring about upsetting thoughts/memories?	
Brooding over things and therefore no longer living my own life to the full?	
Avoiding discussing how I am feeling or coping?	
Avoiding people/isolating myself from others?	
Avoiding being assertive about my own needs?	
Avoiding going out in public, either by myself or with the person experiencing symptoms?	
Avoiding being at home and keeping so busy that I don't have to think about the problem?	
For partners: Avoiding sex or physical intimacy? Perhaps there are fears of overexertion or of causing harm or issues about whether this would be imposing, inappropriate or not wanted at the moment.	

(?) Am I avoiding things in other ways? Write here how you are doing this if this is applicable to you.

....

....

....

Sometimes, some of these questions can be difficult to discuss. If this is the case, you can always decide to discuss it at a later time. This may be the case especially with topics such as sex and intimacy. These are important, though, so try not to ignore things completely.

Remember that at times the avoidance can be quite subtle, for example choosing to steer conversations away from difficult areas that would actually benefit from discussion. Often people fear upsetting the other person or making them feel worse. This can backfire, however, because it leaves issues unaddressed and builds up certain topics as things that 'must not be discussed'.

Overcoming avoidance with clear communication

The only way to overcome avoidance is with openness and honesty. Without openness and honesty, many problems can arise. If you worry about hurting other people's feelings or aren't quite sure how to discuss these things openly, then you might find the workbooks *Being assertive* and *Building relationships* helpful.

Building relationships

You will find it most helpful to make changes slowly. Choose to spend more time together. Start to invite others round. Go out together if you can. Talk to each other – and listen, even if this is difficult.

Find common ground, even if you feel you have drifted apart. Make a joint decision about the level of information to give others about the symptoms. For example, deciding together on a simple one-line reply 'Things are much the same/going well' might be enough for most situations. Here are some practical phrases and strategies you can use to relate differently to each other:

- 'This isn't a good time to talk. Let's talk about it later.'
- Sometimes people need to work through an issue by talking at length. Let them talk – often, no comment is needed. Listen for the main message and then pick up on this point so the person knows you are really listening, e.g. 'It sounds like you feel frustrated/fed up today . . .'
- Offer praise and encouragement to build confidence, e.g. 'I can see such a difference from a month or so ago . . .'
- Actively look for things you can comment on positively.
- Try to find at least three positive things to say every day.

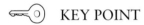 KEY POINT

Clear communication and children

Children may have all sorts of unrealistic fears about possible outcomes if they are kept in the dark. A child may worry that they have caused the problem or fear that their parent or sibling may die or go away as a result of the symptoms. They may blame themselves or become scared of all sorts of consequences. Bearing in mind the age and maturity of the child, try to pitch things at the right level and with sufficient explanation that is helpful for them. If you are uncertain exactly how much to tell them, you might discuss this with your doctor, health worker or the child's schoolteacher or adviser.

Section 3   **Family and friends: helpful and unhelpful responses**

When someone we care about needs our help, we often try to improve things through a range of actions. These might include a range of **helpful** responses that can improve how they and we feel. Sometimes, however – and without meaning to – how we react can become **unhelpful**.

This section of the workbook focuses on both the helpful and possible unhelpful behaviours that we as friends/relatives/carers may do.

Helpful behaviours

Helpful behaviours of relatives and friends can include:
- Finding out about the problem, e.g. by reading the workbooks in this course or other information booklets and getting information from self-help groups and healthcare practitioners. This can equip you with the knowledge and skills you need. You may find the online course at www.livinglifetothefull.com helpful. This is a resource to support users of this book.
- Being there for the person for the long term.
- Being willing to talk and offer support when needed.
- Encouraging the person to put what they are learning in this course into practice.
- Keeping a positive but realistic outlook that change is possible but will take time.
- Realising there are no quick fixes.
- Using your sense of humour to help you and the person you support to cope.
- Planning time for you as well as others.
- Using effective coping responses, such as relaxation techniques, to deal with your feelings of tension.
- Looking after yourself.
- Seeing a healthcare practitioner for advice if you struggle to cope.

(?) Am I doing any other helpful things? Write here what you are doing if this applies to you:

✎

....

....

....

By planning to boost these helpful activities, this can improve how you and those around you feel.

The circle of helpful behaviour

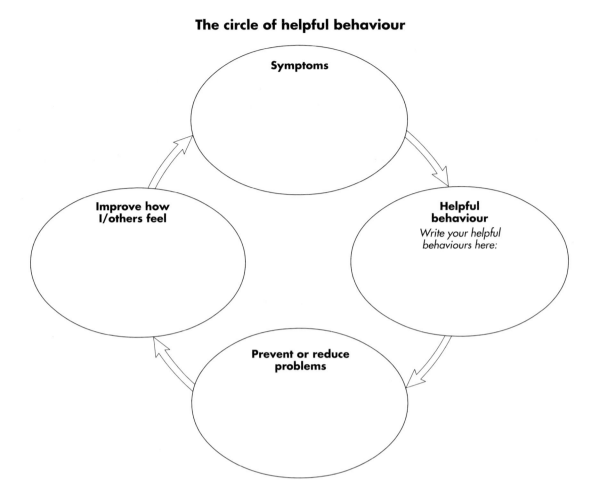

A word of caution: sometimes we can think that a behaviour is helpful when in fact it is part of the problem. Common examples are patterns of excessive drinking, avoidance and reassurance-seeking. Each of these may cause the person to feel better in the short term (which is why they can be mistaken as helpful). However, in the medium or long term, these behaviours backfire and worsen how you or others feel in some way (physically, mentally or in your relationships). In contrast, a hallmark of a truly helpful activity is that it is good for you and often for others as well.

Unhelpful behaviours

Sometimes, friends and family members can act in ways that worsen the situation. These actions are often done with the best of intentions. Sometimes we react out of frustration to let off steam. Although this can make us feel better initially, it can also backfire and create further problems. For example, raising our voice in frustration can make us feel a lot better to begin with but can have a damaging effect on our relationship and leave us feeling guilty.

One way of thinking about this is that sometimes, no matter how helpful something may seem to begin with, if taken to an extreme most responses can backfire. For example, several alcoholic drinks with friends can be part of a nice night out. In contrast, drinking all the time in order to block out feelings becomes an addiction or problem in itself. Another example is that seeking support from others is sensible – a problem shared can really help. But if you find that you are constantly on the phone and feel you cannot cope without talking to others to reassure you, then something that was originally helping has become a problem.

The results of unhelpful behaviours include both immediate and longer-term problems. A **vicious circle of unhelpful behaviour** may result.

Other examples of unhelpful behaviour include:

● Offering 'helpful advice' **all the time**.
● A desire to do **everything** for the person.
● **Constantly** offering reassurance that everything will work out fine ('Of course you'll be OK').
● Overly protecting and suffocating the person by taking away **all** their responsibility and choices.

You can see that the words in bold here make the same point again and again. The motive may be good, and some of these actions may be helpful to some extent. However, taken to extremes, they become unhelpful.

There can be many reasons for us behaving in this way. Often it is due to concern, friendship and love. Sometimes it is the result of anxiety or, occasionally, guilt. Whatever the cause, when we offer too much help and want to do everything for someone else, our actions can backfire and worsen things.

The circle of unhelpful behaviour

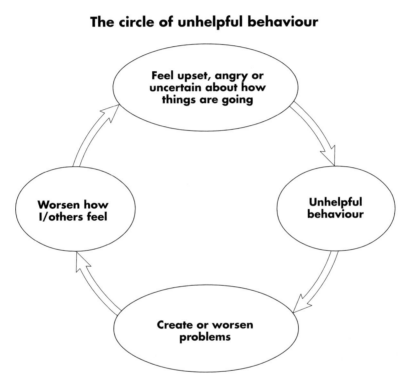

Frustration and anger at healthcare practitioners

It's very common for someone who takes on a supportive or carer role to struggle themselves. Different feelings such as demoralisation, worry, guilt, frustration and even anger can occur. These feelings can spill over into how we talk about healthcare practitioners. It can be tempting to become critical and have very jaundiced views. Most healthcare practitioners are able to offer helpful support to people. However, from time to time even those working in the caring professions may not be able to offer the kind of support that you feel is needed. The danger is that you undermine the support and advice that they can offer if you become critical of them.

But what if I disagree?

Sometimes we have strong opinions about what treatments or investigations are needed. For example, we may have strong opinions about complementary medicine or just not be happy that the current treatment is working. If you find that treatments or investigations are being suggested that you are concerned about, it's important to be aware of how you respond. Try not to persuade the person who has been prescribed medication to suddenly stop it without discussion with their doctor. If you have strong concerns that a treatment is wrong or not needed, it is best for both of you to go along (providing the person who is ill is happy for you to do this) to the doctor to discuss things. What all of you want is the best possible outcome.

Look at the following list. A wide range of different unhelpful behaviours has been summarised here to help you to think about the changes that are happening in your own situation. Tick any activities you have found yourself doing over the past month.

As a friend/family member, am I:	Tick here if you have noticed this, even if only sometimes
Becoming overly protective of the person and wrapping them in cotton wool?	
Taking over all responsibility from the person, e.g. making all the key decisions with no discussion or trying to control every aspect of their life? The result is undermined confidence and often resentment	
Taking over all activities the person used to enjoy or be responsible for so they do not have to 'worry' about them, e.g. household tasks or taking children to school?	
Feeling the need to earn more so the person does not have to work?	
Not allowing the person to be upset or distressed and trying to 'buck them up' all the time?	
Having a go at the person from time to time through frustration or anger?	
Becoming so focused on the distressed person that other people's needs aren't met, e.g. my own needs or the needs of other family members, such as my children?	
Depending on/needing the sufferer to be well and functioning so that they aren't allowed permission to be unwell?	
Talking only about how hard and difficult things are? This contributes to a downward emotional spiral	
Making snap decisions about important issues, e.g. resigning from a job?	
Automatically advising the person not to try treatment approaches because of fears that they may do harm?	
Undermining or criticising healthcare practitioners because they haven't been able to find a cure?	
Ignoring or leaving unaddressed tensions that should be dealt with but are overlooked because of the focus on caring?	
Helping the person to avoid doing things because of fears about what harm might result, e.g. taking over shopping or driving? This then further undermines their confidence	
Constantly reassuring the person in order to allay their anxious fears?	

As a friend/family member, am I:	Tick here if you have noticed this, even if only sometimes
Constantly asking about how they are, which unhelpfully draws attention to illness?	
Introducing the person as 'X, who has this problem', rather than just by their name? You have started seeing the symptoms rather than the person	
Always telling the person to avoid activities because you are concerned about their health, including activities recommended by their healthcare practitioner?	
Speaking for or over the person in social or hospital settings? You tell their story on their behalf even when they are able to themselves	

Write here any other unhelpful behaviours:

✎

....

....

....

(?) **Overall,** what impact do your unhelpful behaviours have on you both?

✎

....

....

....

The problem is that these responses can quickly become a habit, where the same patterns are repeated again and again.

Wrapping the person in cotton wool

Offering extra special attention and support can also become unhelpful. The relationship may feel suffocating and frustrating. The person can end up feeling as though you are treating them like a child. Arguments and little irritations build up and are upsetting for everyone. Although we mean well, our actions can actually undermine our relationship. When trying to cope with symptoms, it is important to encourage the person to keep as active as possible within the confines of how they feel. If we take responsibility for doing everything for the person, the danger is that they will not be as active as they could be and we create unnecessary dependency.

EXAMPLE

Becoming overly protective

Background: after a mild heart attack, Patrick is convinced that his heart is not working properly. As a result, he constantly feels anxious and is preoccupied with his illness. He feels physically tense and cannot sleep. He has stopped any activities that he fears may bring on a heart attack, such as doing exercise and making love with his wife. He pays especial attention to the speed of his pulse and to any twinges of pain in his chest, whatever the cause. He has become so anxious about his pulse that he takes it all the time. His doctor has advised him that he needs to do some exercise in order to stay fit. Patrick now feels that he is unable to do any exercise at all, even though physically it is recommended as part of his heart recovery programme. He is scared of doing things that raise his heart rate, just in case it is dangerous.

Situation: Patrick and his wife Joyce are walking in the park half a mile from home. This is the first time he has been so far from home. He begins to become aware of his heart beating and starts to feel his pulse. His wife anxiously asks him how he feels and tells him to sit down on a bench. She leaves her mobile phone with him and walks home quickly to get the car. When she gets back, he is looking tense and sweaty. She drives him home and puts him to bed. After that, she decides 'That's the last time we go for a walk. He's much too ill for that.'

Patrick's key problems are:

● **Avoidance:** he becomes scared and stops walking. He also does various things to feel safer. These so-called safety behaviours include looking for reassurance from Joyce, seeking excessive checks from his doctor, and feeling his pulse all the time.

● **How Joyce's behaviour worsens things:** Joyce cares for and wants to protect Patrick. However, because Joyce wraps him in cotton wool, Patrick is unable to do the cardiac rehabilitation package recommended by his doctor.

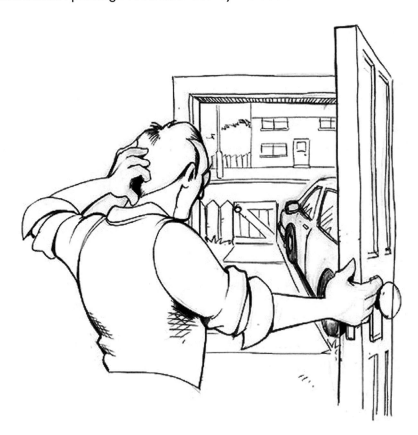

This is bad for Patrick physically. Even worse, though, is that Joyce and Patrick are building up each other's fears. Patrick is in danger of not being able to go anywhere – walks, holidays or shopping. If Joyce takes over all these responsibilities, it will also be too hard for her. These sorts of things are best shared. In fact, by encouraging Patrick to slowly but surely pace an increase in his activity, he could rebuild his confidence in doing things. Joyce's lack of confidence may prevent this. She needs to build her confidence that Patrick will be fine if he increases his activity slowly but surely. Joyce has done this with the best intentions, but she just hasn't thought through the longer-term consequences.

Staying well ourselves

When we support others, we also need to look after ourselves and allow time and space for our own needs. Depression and stress are very common among carers. The danger is that we are so busy offering support that we have no time for ourselves.

Helpful responses to look after ourselves include:

- Open discussion of your own stress as an issue, e.g. with your own doctor or perhaps within a carer support group.
- Taking short breaks, holidays or weekends away with others.
- Planning 'me time', such as hobbies and classes.
- Attending relaxation or stress-management classes or carer support groups.
- Seeing your own doctor to discuss the need for additional treatment and support.

Problem actions and activities we need to be aware of

Although we try to cope as best we can, sometimes some of our ways of reacting can backfire and worsen the situation. The following are some common unhelpful behaviours that we may use in order to help ourselves cope.

As a friend/family member, am I trying to cope by:	Tick here if you have noticed this, even if only sometimes
Throwing myself into doing things so there are no opportunities to stop, think and reflect?	
Pushing others away and being verbally or physically threatening or rude to them?	
Becoming very demanding of others?	
Looking to others to make decisions or sort out problems for me?	
Drinking more alcohol than I should in order to block how I feel?	
Using medication differently to how it is prescribed in order to improve how I feel or help me sleep, e.g. taking extra doses?	
Eating too much ('comfort eating') or overeating so much that it becomes bingeing?	

As a friend/family member, am I trying to cope by:	Tick here if you have noticed this, even if only sometimes
Trying to spend my way out of how I feel by going shopping ('retail therapy')?	
Deliberately harming myself because of frustration or desperation or in order to reduce tension?	
Taking part in risk-taking actions, e.g. crossing the road without looking or gambling using money I don't really have?	

The next section provides some hints and tips to help you begin to reduce any unhelpful behaviours.

Section 4 Breaking the vicious circles and building helpful behaviours

To successfully plan a reduction in unhelpful behaviours or to increase helpful behaviours, you need to have a clear plan.

Do:
- Produce a plan to slowly alter what you do in a step-by-step way.
- Plan to alter only one key response over the next week. Do this one step at a time until you reach your eventual goal.
- Write down your plan in detail so that are able to put it into practice this week.

Don't:
- Choose something a target that is too ambitious.
- Try to alter too many things all at once.
- Be very negative and think 'Nothing can be done. What's the point? It's a waste of time.' (Instead, try to experiment to find out whether this negative thinking is accurate or helpful.)

Reducing unhelpful behaviours

Throwing yourself into doing things for the person all the time; wrapping the person in cotton wool	You need a balance of time for you, while still offering appropriate support for the person. Plan a slow reduction in this 'over-caring' activity. Explain to the person why you are doing this so that it doesn't come out of the blue. There will be two benefits: doing this will give you some 'me time' and will prevent the person from feeling suffocated and controlled. They may have become used to and dependent on this close level of support; perhaps you have too. You may need to explore new hobbies and interests. They may need to make some changes too. The key is communication and getting the right balance that suits you both
Being critical or rude towards or about the person or others who ask about how they or you are	What situations or people bring this on? Are you testing out their friendship or love for you? You may well be angry at the person you are supporting for not getting better, for not trying or just for being ill. We may know that these reactions aren't logical, but we can feel angry nonetheless. Sometimes we may want to create a reason that allows us to separate or withdraw. What is needed here is time, space and communication. Plan some gaps. Do some things apart. Look at ways of rebuilding your relationship or friendship, perhaps by using the workbook *Building relationships*

Being overly aware of and excessively checking for symptoms of ill health or distress	If you find that you are constantly asking the person how they feel or commenting about how they look, try to break this habit by becoming aware that this is a problem. Set yourself limits on how often you ask these questions, and try to gradually reduce this. That does not mean you stop talking completely – just that the topic of conversation can change from illness to other issues, such as the weather or football. If you find you ask about symptoms and then suddenly remember that this is unhelpful, try to move to another topic as soon as possible. The person you are supporting might be dependent on this sort of reassurance and may become anxious if you stop offering this. It is important to explain why you are doing this and the intention behind it. The person you care for may feel more anxious for a time, so you may need to agree jointly the right pace that allows this change to occur. They might find it helpful to read the workbook *Overcoming reduced activity and avoidance*. Similarly, if they constantly look for reassurance, try to reduce this slowly (by agreement) to a more helpful and appropriate level

Building helpful behaviours and reducing unhelpful behaviours

The seven-step plan below can help you to plan to do things differently. Think about how you can begin to tackle the problems you face in your own life. This may be:
- To reduce any unhelpful behaviour.
- To build up a helpful behaviour.

You will already have an idea of the different activities you are doing from the checklists you have completed in this workbook. In fact, if you try to change everything at once, you will set yourself up to fail. The important first step is to identify a **single** initial target area that you can focus on. This is particularly important if you have ticked a number of boxes in the checklists. You need to decide which **one** area to focus on to start with. This means putting any other areas to one side for the time being.

If you get stuck, have a look at the examples on pages 19–20. More detailed examples are given in the workbooks *Practical problem-solving* and *Overcoming reduced activity and avoidance*.

Step 1: identify and define the problem as precisely as possible
Write the problem here:

✎

....

....

....

(?) Is this clear and focused?   Yes ☐   No ☐

If no, rewrite it here so that it is clear and focused:

✎

....

....

....

Step 2: think of as many solutions as possible in order to achieve your initial goal

It may be that the thought of making changes seems daunting or impossible. There are all sorts of different ways to tackle the various problems and issues you face. Likewise, there are all sorts of ways to build up helpful behaviours. To help you get a range of possible solutions, use an approach called **brainstorming**.

In brainstorming, try to think broadly and be creative in your answers. You want to come up with as many ideas as possible. Among these ideas, you hope to be able to identify a realistic, practical and achievable solution. The more solutions that are generated, the more likely it is that a good one will emerge. Completely wacky ideas should be included, even if you would never choose them in practice. This can help you to adopt a flexible approach to the issue.

Useful questions to help you think up a good first step include:

- What advice would I give a friend who was trying to tackle the same problem? (Sometimes we can think of solutions more easily for others than for ourselves.)
- What ridiculous solutions can I include, as well as the more sensible ideas?
- What helpful ideas would others (e.g. family, friends or work colleagues) suggest?
- How could I look at the solutions facing me differently? (For example, what would you have said before you felt like this, or what might you say about the situation say in five years' time?)
- What approaches have I tried in the past in similar circumstances?

If you feel stuck, doing this task with someone you trust can be helpful sometimes.

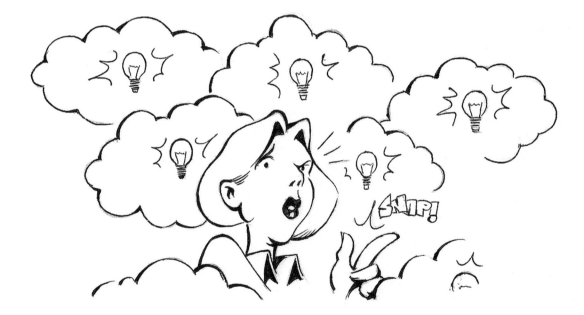

The purpose of brainstorming is to try to come up with as many ideas as possible. Try to create as many ideas as you can. If this proves difficult, try to think of some bizarre ideas first to help get the ideas flowing.

Possible options (including ridiculous ideas first) are:

....

....

....

....

....

....

....

....

....

....

....

....

Step 3: look at the advantages and disadvantages of each possible solution

My suggestions	Advantages	Disadvantages

Step 4: choose one of the solutions

Look at your own responses in Step 3. From these, you should choose a solution.

What you are looking for most often is to find a **step-by step** approach where no step seems too large. The sort of solution you are looking for is, therefore, something that gets you moving in the right direction. This should be small enough to be possible but big enough to move you forwards. Write your solution here:

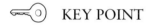

....

....

....

Your solution should be an option that fulfils the following criteria:

Is it **useful** for changing how you are?	Yes ☐	No ☐
Is it a **clear task**, so you will know when you have done it?	Yes ☐	No ☐
Is it something that is realistic, practical and achievable?	Yes ☐	No ☐

Step 5: plan the steps needed to carry out the solution

Write down the practical steps needed to carry out your plan. Try to be very specific so that you know **what** you are going to do and **when** you are going to do it.

KEY POINT

You need to generate a clear plan that will help you to decide exactly what you are going to do and when you are going to do it. It is useful to **write down** the steps needed to carry out your solution. This will help you to plan what to do and will allow you to predict possible problems that might arise. Remember to build into your plan some thought about what you will do if the plan doesn't succeed fully.

My plan (include ways of tackling any possible blocks that might get in the way):

✎

....

....

....

....

....

....

....

....

....

....

....

....

....

....

....

....

....

....

This is the **key part** of the problem-solving process. Be as precise as possible in your plan.

Next, apply the **questions for effective change** to your plan in order to check how practical and achievable it is. Is my plan one that:

Will be useful for understanding or changing how I am?	Yes ☐	No ☐
Is a specific task, so that I will know when I have done it?	Yes ☐	No ☐
Is realistic, practical and achievable?	Yes ☐	No ☐
Makes clear what I am going to do and when I am going to do it?	Yes ☐	No ☐
Is an activity that won't be easily blocked or prevented by practical problems?	Yes ☐	No ☐
Will help me to learn useful things, even if it doesn't work out perfectly?	Yes ☐	No ☐

You should be able to answer yes to each of these questions. If your current plan has failed on one of the questions, try to change or alter things so that any poorly planned aspects are improved.

Note: part of this planning phase should include planning what you will do if your initial plan doesn't work out fully. What if it doesn't work out? Write your plan here:

✎

....

....

....

Step 6: carry out the plan

Pay attention to your thoughts about what will happen before, during and after you have completed your plan.

(task) Write down any extreme and unhelpful thoughts you noticed. Record how much you believed them at the time, from 0% (not at all) to 100% (fully).

My thought(s):

✎

....

....

....

I believed this   % **before** the task.

I believed this   % **during** the task.

I believed this   % **after** the task.

Record how anxious you felt at the time, from 0% (not at all) to 100% (maximum possible anxiety).

My level of anxiety: % **before** the task.

My level of anxiety: % **during** the task.

My level of anxiety: % **after** the task.

The best way to undermine anxious fears is to act against them.

Step 7: review the outcome

My review – write what happened here:

✎

....

....

....

Was the approach successful?	Yes ☐	No ☐
Did it improve things?	Yes ☐	No ☐
Were there any disadvantages to using this approach?	Yes ☐	No ☐

(?) What have I learned from doing this? Write down any helpful lessons or information you have learned from what happened. If things didn't go quite as you hoped, try to learn from this. How could you make things different during your next attempt to tackle the problem?

✎

....

....

....

Try to learn from any mistakes and keep practising so that using this approach becomes second nature whenever you face a problem.

Workbook summary

In this workbook you have learned:
- What this course is about and how the person is using it.
- How best to help and communicate effectively with the person.
- Helpful and unhelpful things you can do so that you can offer effective support.
- How to look after yourself and stay well.

Putting into practice what you have learned

Reflect on the seven-step plan and consider how you can:
- Reduce one **unhelpful behaviour** or area of **avoidance** over the next week.
- Plan to build upon one **helpful response** this week.

Remember: do not try to do everything all at once. Instead, plan out what to do at a pace that is right for you. Discuss this with a friend or your healthcare practitioner if you are stuck or unsure about what to do.

Where to get more help

You may find the course content at www.livinglifetothefull.com helpful. This is the companion support site for users of this book and their carers and friends. A wide range of local carer supports are also available. Ask your GP or local social services for information.

Acknowledgements

Thank you to Marie Chellingsworth, Catriona Kent, Nicky Dummett and Alison Williams for comments on this workbook. Illustrations are by Keith Chan and are reproduced by permission of Dr Chris Williams.

My notes

....

....

....

....

....

....

....

....

....

....

....

....

....

....

....

....

....

....

....

....

....

....

....

....

....

My notes

....

....

Noticing and changing extreme and unhelpful thinking

Dr Chris Williams

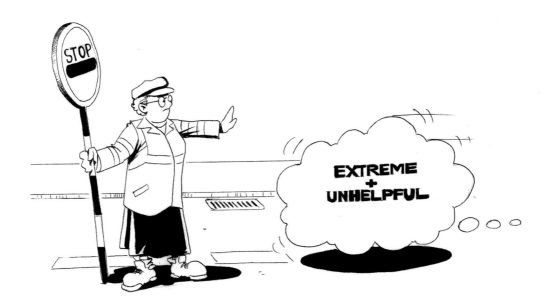

A Five Areas Approach
Helping you to help yourself
www.livinglifetothefull.com

Section 1   **Introduction**

When we feel unwell we often start to notice:
- Anxious fears, which make us feel tense and stressed.
- Unhappy negative thoughts, which make us feel low and sad.
- Frustrated angry thoughts at ourselves, our situation and sometimes other people, such as our friends and relatives.

We may have all sorts of unhelpful thoughts about how we feel, our current situation and our future outlook.

In this workbook you will learn how to:
- Notice patterns of extreme and unhelpful thinking that worsen how you feel.
- Change extreme and unhelpful thinking.
- Experiment and test out your thinking.
- Come up with more balanced and helpful thoughts.
- Tackle difficulties, such as what to do if thoughts go round and round in your head.

The first step in changing unhelpful thinking is to start noticing how **common** it is in your own life. Frustration, anger, distress, shame, guilt and feeling down are often linked to the following unhelpful patterns of thinking:

Unhelpful thinking style	Typical thoughts	Tick if you have noticed this thinking style recently, even if only sometimes
Bias against myself	I'm very self-critical I overlook my strengths I see myself as not coping I don't recognise my achievements	
Putting a negative slant on things (negative mental filter)	I see things through dark-tinted glasses I see the glass as being half empty rather than half full Whatever I've done in the week, it's never enough to give me a sense of achievement I tend to focus on the bad side of everyday situations	
Having a gloomy view of the future (make negative predictions)	I think that things will stay bad or get even worse I tend to predict that things will go wrong If one thing goes wrong, I often predict that everything will go wrong I'm always looking for the next thing to fail	

Unhelpful thinking style	Typical thoughts	Tick if you have noticed this thinking style recently, even if only sometimes
Jumping to the very worst conclusion (catastrophising)	I tend to predict that the very worst outcome will happen I often think that I will fail terribly badly	
Having a negative view about how others see me (mind-reading)	I mind-read what others think of me I often think that others don't like me or think badly of me without evidence	
Unfairly taking responsibility for things	I think I should take the blame if things go wrong I feel guilty about things that are not really my fault I think I'm responsible for everyone else	
Making extreme statements/rules	I use the words 'always' and 'never' a lot to summarise things If one bad thing happens to me, I often say 'Just typical!' because it seems this always happens I make myself a lot of 'must', 'should', 'ought' and 'got to' rules I believe I must push myself to do things well	

All of these are examples of extreme thinking. Often we believe these thoughts just because they 'feel' true as a result of how we're feeling in ourselves. We may forget to check out how true these thoughts really are.

This doesn't mean that:

- You think like this **all** the time.
- You have to notice **all** of the unhelpful thinking styles.

Almost everyone has these sorts of thoughts each and every day. They are often present and can affect how we feel.

How do these patterns of thinking affect us?

Usually when we notice these thoughts, we feel a little upset but then quickly dismiss the thought and carry on with life.

However, there are times in life when we are more prone to these thoughts and find them harder to dismiss. For example, in difficult times or if we are distressed, we typically notice these thoughts more often. We may dwell on them more than usual and find it harder to dismiss them and move on.

What we think can have a powerful impact on us. It affects how we **feel** and what we **do**.

The unhelpful thinking styles lead to:

- **Mood changes:** you may become more down, guilty, upset, anxious, ashamed, stressed or angry.
- **Behaviour changes:** by **reducing** or **stopping** what we do or causing us to **avoid** things that make us feel anxious. Finally, we may start to act in **unhelpful** ways that end up backfiring and worsen how we feel. An example is drinking too much alcohol: although we may think this helps, in the longer term it backfires and can become part of the problem.

The result is that these unhelpful thinking styles act to worsen how you feel.

We have already seen two examples: John's wallet in the workbook *Starting out* (page 9) and walking down the street in the workbook *Understanding why I feel as I do* (page 7). These show that how we interpret events can affect how we feel and what we do.

 Look at the links between our thoughts, feelings and behaviour for these two examples. You will see in the last column a suggestion that stopping, thinking and reflecting could really help you get a different perspective before you feel worse.

(e.g.) EXAMPLE

Situation	Unhelpful thinking style	Altered feelings	Altered behaviour
You are walking down the road and someone you know walks past and says nothing. They don't smile or meet your eye; they just walk by. **Thought:** 'There's poor Paul – he looks really distracted and upset. I hope he's OK'	Normal concern for others, no unhelpful thinking styles	Concern for Paul	Turns round and catches up with Paul to say hello. Paul looks a little surprised to begin with and says he didn't see you. You get chatting and have a really helpful talk. At the end, you both agree to meet for lunch after the shopping to catch up **Stop, think and reflect:** 'I'm really pleased I spoke to him. He is feeling upset. It was nice to talk – and he seemed pleased too. He suggested we meet up for lunch, which is good because it says to me that he wants to see me'
You are walking down the road and someone you know walks past and says nothing. They don't smile or meet your eye; they just walk by. **Thought:** 'They don't like me'	Mind-reading they don't like you, jump to the worst conclusion, bias against yourself	Low, down, upset; anxious in case you meet again Feel so down you just go home. Avoid them in future	**Stop, think and reflect:** 'I never checked out that this was the real reason. Maybe they just didn't see me'
John comes home from shopping and realises with a start that he cannot find his wallet. **Thought:** 'It's been stolen – the thieves will be buying goods all over the place with my money!'	Catastrophic thinking	Very anxious, on edge, scared of the consequences	Immediately phones and cancels his credit cards Later finds them in his coat pocket **Stop, think and reflect:** 'I've lost them before and then found them. I'll have a good look before cancelling them'

| You are at the checkout of the supermarket and hear someone behind you tut as you pack your bags. **Thought:** 'I'm being too slow. They're annoyed at me' | Bias against yourself (blame yourself), mind-reading | Anxiety, perhaps anger – 'How dare they?' | If **anxious**, maybe speed up packing, fumble, start to drop things, make all sorts of apologies
If **angry**, perhaps slow down the packing, stare at them or pass a sarcastic comment

Stop, think and reflect: 'Maybe they were tutting at something else. Maybe they'd forgotten to pick up their apples. Maybe their teeth don't fit!' |
| Harvinder has had fears of going shopping for over six months and these are gradually getting worse. He is now in the middle of a long queue at the supermarket. **Thought:** 'I'm going to collapse and pass out' | Catastrophic thinking | Anxiety, physical symptoms of faster heart rate and rapid breathing | **Avoidance:** tending to avoid supermarkets and shopping only when it is quieter
Unhelpful behaviours: walks around the store faster than usual and leaves the store quickly in order to sit down
Stop, think and reflect: 'I have never collapsed. I know that panic can make people feel like this' |

 KEY POINT

The different unhelpful thinking styles are common patterns of thinking that can worsen how you feel and affect what you do. They are more common than you may expect at times of distress. Thinking in these extreme ways means that you look at only part of the picture. Because of this, these thinking styles are often not true.

Mental pictures/images

Another way that we think is as a mental picture. Some (but not all) people notice mental pictures or images in their mind from time to time. Images are a form of thought. They may be still images (like a photograph) or moving images (like a video). Images may be in black and white or in colour.

Images may include:

● Predictions of the **future**, e.g. worsening symptoms.
● Memories of **past** events, e.g. previous significant problems.
● Thoughts about things that are **currently** happening, e.g. images of how we think others see us.

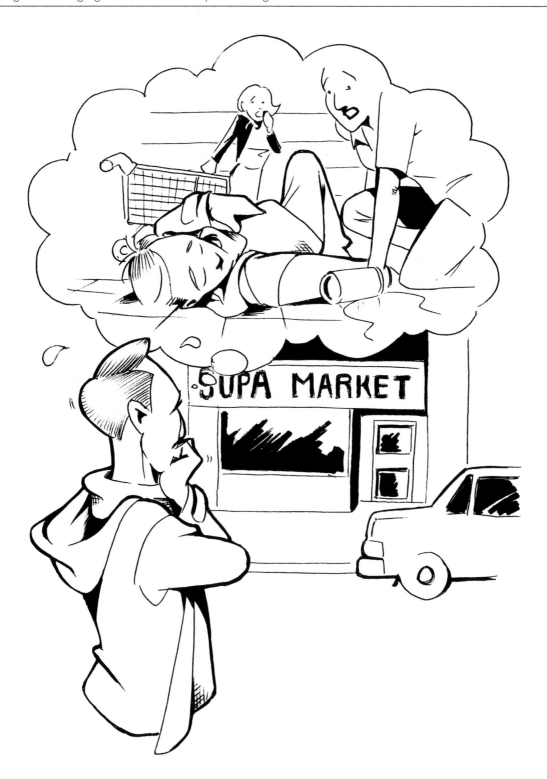

Images can also show any of the unhelpful thinking styles. Which thinking styles are shown in the image above?

The next step is to practise ways of **noticing** extreme and unhelpful thinking. This is the first and most important step in beginning to change how you think. Once you can notice these patterns in your thinking, you can step back and choose not to get caught up in these thinking patterns.

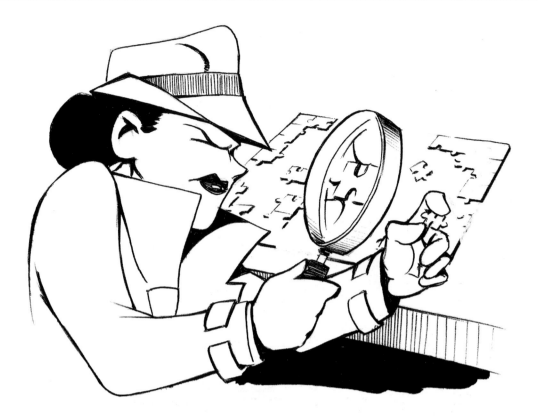

To get used to noticing these sorts of thought, you will need to act like a **thought detective** by carrying out a **thought review** – an investigation of times when your mood alters unhelpfully.

Section 2   Noticing extreme and unhelpful thinking

The examples on the following pages will help you begin to see how extreme thinking may affect how you feel and what you do. Try to **act like a detective** to piece together bit by bit the factors that led up to you feeling worse.

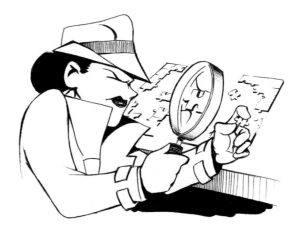

Hint: in order to identify extreme or unhelpful thinking, try to watch for times when you suddenly feel worse, e.g. physically worse, sadder, or more anxious, upset, guilty or angry. Then ask yourself: 'What went through my mind then?'

The following questions can help Anne work out for herself the five areas that may be linked to feeling worse. It helps her look in detail at:

- The situation, relationship or practical problems that occurred.
- The altered thinking, such as extreme or unhelpful thinking styles.
- Altered feelings (also called mood or emotions).
- Altered physical symptoms.
- Finally, the altered behaviour that occurred, such as reduced activity, avoidance or starting to do unhelpful behaviours.

 EXAMPLE

Anne's thought investigation of a time when she has felt worse

Background: Anne has been feeling low for much of the year, since her brother and his family moved away. Although they talk by phone, it isn't the same. She misses her nephew Tom and her niece Sarah. Her sister Mary lives locally and drops in occasionally for a cup of tea.

For the past few months, Anne has been feeling increasingly low and upset. She has become more and more isolated and sits crying, looking at photos of Tom and Sarah. She is doing far less than usual. She has asked her sister Mary not to visit her because she worries what Mary will think of her. She worries that often she hasn't tidied up and is aware the flat looks a mess.

The specific situation when Anne feels worse:

Situation: it's 10 a.m. on Tuesday. Anne has only just got up. The doorbell rings – it's Mary, who has come by unexpectedly.

Thinking: 'Oh no! I always look awful. She'll think I'm not coping.'

Feelings: ashamed, low and sad.

Physical symptoms: blushed, felt a feeling of tension and pain, and went hot.

Behaviour: acted quite flustered, avoided eye contact, made an excuse after ten minutes and lied by saying I had a doctor's appointment.

Her main problems here are:
- **Unhelpful thinking style:** mind-reading what Mary will think.
- **Unhelpful behaviour:** her shame leads her to lie to her sister – something she feels even more ashamed about later.

Anne writes her reactions into all five areas.

Anne's reaction to Mary's visit

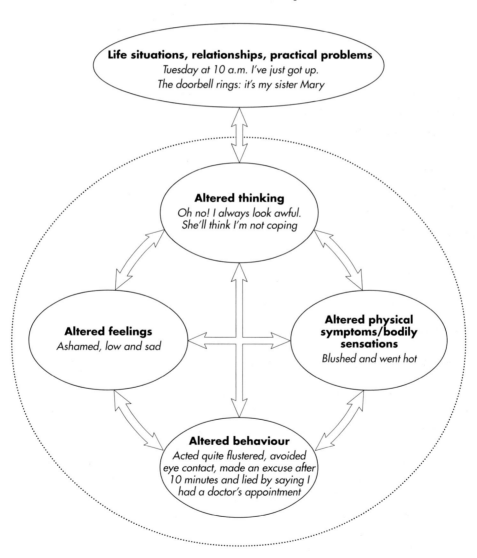

Think about Anne's reaction to the situation. How do Anne's thoughts and interpretation of what happened tie in to how she felt and what she did?

EXAMPLE

Harvinder's thought investigation of a time when he has felt worse

Background: Harvinder has occasional panic attacks when he is in large shops such as supermarkets. These attacks began out of the blue five years ago. Since then, he has found it increasingly difficult to go into large shops. Instead, he mostly visits smaller shops at quiet times of day or arranges Internet shopping delivery. Sometimes he asks others to do the shopping for him.

The specific situation when Harvinder feels worse:

Harvinder had decided he must go to the supermarket.

- **Situation:** as he got near the door of the shop.

- **Physical:** his heart was pumping heavily; he also felt hot, a little sweaty and tense.

- **Feelings:** anxious.

- **Thinking:** 'Oh no! I'm not feeling good. It might happen.'

- **Behaviour:** walks a little faster and grabs a trolley to find the things he needs quickly.

Harvinder just entering the shop

Life situations, relationships, practical problems
Gets near the door of the shop

Altered thinking
Oh no! I'm not feeling good. It might happen

Altered feelings
Anxious

Altered physical symptoms/bodily sensations
Heart pumping, hot, a little sweaty and tense

Altered behaviour
Walks faster and grabs a trolley

Note: the first thing Harvinder notices is his heart and breathing. This then starts him worrying about what will happen.

Harvinder then enters the shop:

- **Situation:** as he continues shopping, things quickly get worse.

- **Physical:** his heart is now really pumping heavily. He is overbreathing, with rapid shallow breaths, and he feels physically ill, hot and dizzy.

- **Feelings:** his sense of fear and tension has worsened. He now feels very anxious, almost terrified and very panicky.

- **Thinking:** 'I'm going to suffocate – I can't catch my breath. I've got to get out of here.'

- **Behaviour:** he starts to grip on to the trolley and walks even faster. He eventually drops everything and walks rapidly to the door. He leaves the supermarket and sits down. After ten minutes he feels better but promises himself 'Never again!'

His main problems here are:
- **Unhelpful thinking style:** catastrophic fears that he will suffocate.
- **Avoidance:** he becomes scared and does various things to make himself feel safer. These so-called safety behaviours include walking faster, gripping the trolley, and eventually leaving and sitting down.

Harvinder inside the shop

Life situations, relationships, practical problems
Things quickly get worse, feel ill

Altered thinking
*I'm going to suffocate –
I can't catch my breath, I've
got to get out of here*

Altered feelings
*Fear and tension
Highly anxious
Panicky*

**Altered physical
symptoms/bodily
sensations**
*Heart and breathing +++
Ill, hot and dizzy*

Altered behaviour
*Grips trolley, walks faster,
grabs a trolley
Leaves and sits down*

KEY POINT

What you need to know about anxiety

One of the common reactions in anxiety is the so-called **fight or flight adrenalin response**. Feelings of **mental tension** can also cause **physical tension** in your muscles and joints. This may cause feelings of shakiness, pain, weakness or tiredness. It can be surprising how tiring anxiety can be, and some people may feel completely exhausted when they have felt anxious for a time. This muscle tension can cause problems such as tension headaches, stomach or chest pains. Sensations of being hot, cold, sweaty or clammy are common. The heart may seem to be racing and you may feel fuzzy-headed or disconnected from things.

Common physical symptoms of high anxiety

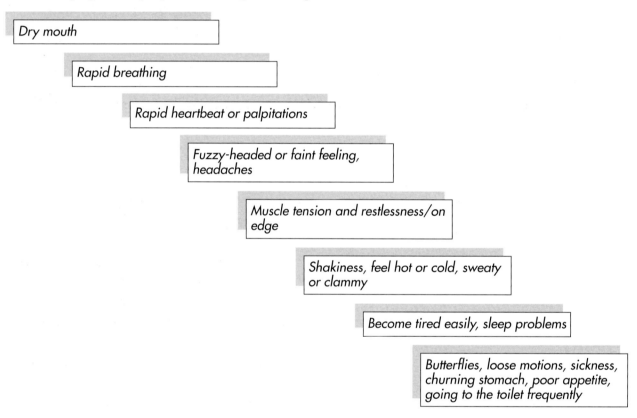

Dry mouth

Rapid breathing

Rapid heartbeat or palpitations

Fuzzy-headed or faint feeling, headaches

Muscle tension and restlessness/on edge

Shakiness, feel hot or cold, sweaty or clammy

Become tired easily, sleep problems

Butterflies, loose motions, sickness, churning stomach, poor appetite, going to the toilet frequently

What causes these physical symptoms?

Our bodies react to extreme and unhelpful frightening thoughts just as they would to a physical danger. The **fight or flight adrenalin response** creates all of the symptoms described above. The heart rate and breathing speed up so that the muscles are ready to react to defend ourselves or run away. This is very useful when the danger is real. Think about a time when you have had a sudden shock – perhaps you stepped into the road when a car was coming and didn't realise until you heard the car horn. Your body releases adrenalin, which makes your heart beat faster. The fight or flight adrenalin response causes the person to pay particular attention to any potential threats around them. There may be other physical responses, such as feeling sweaty or restless and tense. Blood is pumped faster around the body so that the muscles are ready to react. Breathing may speed up to allow more oxygen to get to the muscles. Sometimes rapid breathing continues long enough to cause a state of anxious overbreathing – also known as **hyperventilation.**

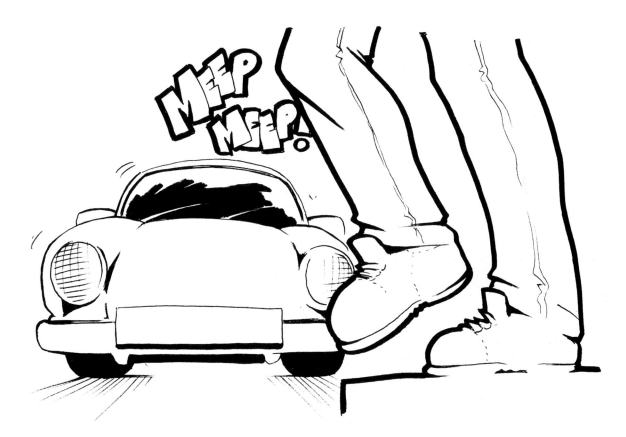

How do these physical changes and our scary catastrophic fears relate to each other?

The fight or flight adrenalin response causes us to pay particular attention to any potential threats around us. Each of us will focus on different threats that are especially scary for us. For example, the experience of a very rapid heart or chest pain in panic may reinforce the fear 'I'm having a heart attack'. Feelings of dizziness and blurred vision caused by overbreathing can reinforce the fear 'I'm about to faint or collapse' or 'I'm having a stroke'. Also, overbreathing with rapid shallow breaths actually causes us to feel even more breathless. This can explain why Harvinder felt as he did.

It is important to recognise that although these sensations are unpleasant, **they are not harmful.**

Two common difficulties

Many people try to deal with their extreme and unhelpful thoughts by using two main strategies. These are both ineffective and can backfire. People often either **try not to think about** the thoughts or **think too much** about them, by analysing the issue in detail to the exclusion of other things. It's easy to understand why we would try so hard to rid ourselves of these extreme and unhelpful thoughts, but it is important to realise that these two techniques are not useful in doing this.

Trying hard not to think about things

Because worrying thoughts focus on topics that are distressing, you may try hard **not** to think about the thoughts. Is this an effective strategy?

EXPERIMENT

In order to see whether trying hard not to think worrying thoughts works, try this practical experiment. Try as hard as you can **not** to think about the following object. Try very hard for the next 30 seconds not to think about a white polar bear.

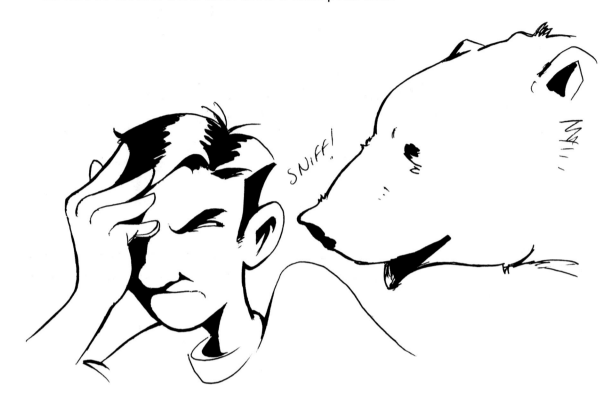

After you have done this, think about what happened. Was it easy to **not think** about the bear, or did it take a lot of effort? You may have noticed that trying hard not to think about it actually made it worse. Alternatively, you may have spent a lot of mental effort trying hard to think about something else such as a **black** polar bear instead. For many people, trying hard to ignore their upsetting thoughts and not think about them doesn't work and may actually worsen the problem. This can be mentally exhausting.

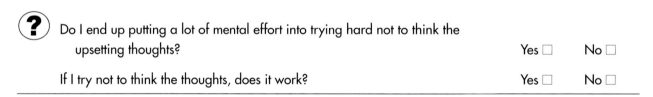

Do I end up putting a lot of mental effort into trying hard not to think the upsetting thoughts?   Yes ☐   No ☐

If I try not to think the thoughts, does it work?   Yes ☐   No ☐

If you think this applies only to you or even that this is not relevant, why not ask a friend or family member to try the experiment too. Experiments can be a really important way of testing out new ideas.

You will find out ways of overcoming this problem in Section 5 of this workbook.

Rumination: going over the same things again and again in your mind

A second common response is to try to **think your way out of the situation** by overanalysing any concerns in great detail. This is well beyond helpfully thinking things through. The result is that the same spiral of thoughts goes round and round in your head. This approach usually isn't effective.

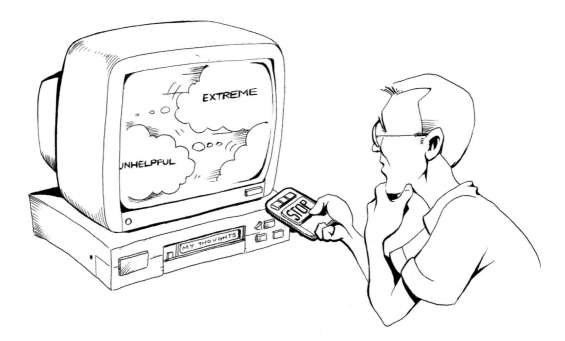

It is far more effective to just **let the thoughts be – don't get caught up in them**. Accept that you have these worries and that you cannot think your way through them. See Section 4 for ways of overcoming such thinking.

Section 3   **Completing your own thought review**

Now you have an opportunity to play thought detective by looking in detail at a specific time when you have felt worse.

   First, try to really think yourself back into a situation in the past few days when you felt worse. To begin with, **don't choose a time when you have felt very distressed**. Instead, pick an occasion when you have noticed **some** worsening upset, tension, symptoms, anger or guilt. Try to slow down as you think back through the situation so that you are as accurate as you can be. Try to stop, think and reflect as you consider the five different areas that can be affected.

Before you start: what to do if you find it is difficult even thinking about the upsetting situation

Sometimes it can feel distressing going back over a time when we have felt worse. That is why it is important to begin by choosing a time that is not so distressing that just looking at it in depth will make you feel too upset. The whole process here aims to empower you to change such thoughts and to feel less distressed. Sometimes our concerns, worries and fears can feel terrifying and too much to look at all in one go. If this is the case for you, the key is to start practising this approach slowly, beginning with less upsetting thoughts. Start to notice the thoughts that link in with you feeling **somewhat or moderately upset**. Don't go for the most distressing and upsetting times immediately. Work with your moderately upsetting thoughts first and use the rest of the workbook to practise changing these. You can slowly work up to more upsetting thoughts later when you are feeling more confident.

 Use the blank five areas diagram on page 17 to go through what you noticed in each of the five areas. Think about:

- **The situation:** where were you? What time of day was it? Who else was there? What was said? What happened? Write this into Box 1.

- **Altered thinking:** what went through your mind at the time? How did you see yourself and how you were coping (bias against yourself)? What did you predict was the worst thing that could happen (catastrophic thinking)? How did you think others saw you (mind-reading)? What did you think about your own body, behaviour or performance? Were there any painful memories from the past? Did you notice any images or pictures in your mind (images can have a powerful impact on how you feel)? Write down any thoughts you notice into Box 2. **Underline** the most upsetting thought.

- **Altered feeling:** how did you feel emotionally at the time? Were you anxious, ashamed, depressed, angry or guilty? Write these into Box 3.

- **Altered physical symptoms:** write these into Box 4. A wide range of physical reactions may occur, such as muscle tension, jitteriness or pain. There may be a wide range of anxiety-related symptoms, e.g. rapid heart and breathing, feeling hot, sweaty and clammy. There may be low mood, with feelings of low energy, pressure or pain.

- **Altered behaviour:** write these into Box 5. Remember altered behaviour can include:
  - **Helpful responses** that can improve how you and/or others feel.
  - **Reduced activity**, where you reduce or stop doing what you had planned to do.
  - **Avoidance**, where you suddenly feel anxious and avoid doing something or going somewhere.
  - **Unhelpful behaviours**, where you try to block how you feel by acting in ways that may make you feel better in the short term but backfire in the longer term.

My five areas thought review of a time when I felt worse

Write in your experiences in all five areas:

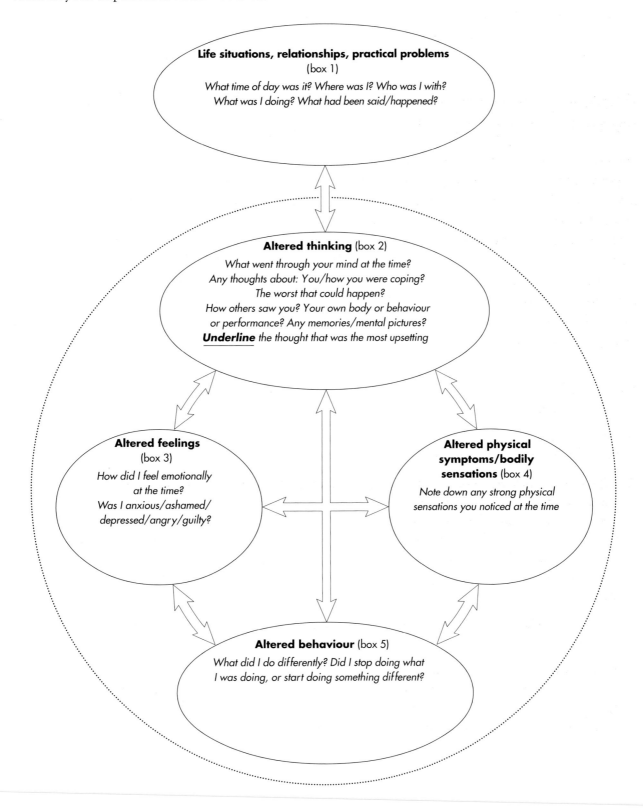

Now that you have finished, re-read your answers. As you do this, try to apply what you know about the **five areas assessment** model to see how each of these areas might have played a part in affecting how you felt. The five areas model shows that **what a person thinks** about a situation or problem may **affect how they feel** physically and emotionally and may lead them to alter **what they do** (altered behaviour).

● What you think affects **how** you feel.
● What you think affects **what** you do.

 Does your thought review show this?   Yes ☐   No ☐

You will find a blank five areas assessment sheet at the end of this workbook. Copy this so you can practise the approach.

At first, many people find it quite difficult to notice their unhelpful thinking. Carrying out this sort of thought review can help you to practise how to do this. Over time you will find that this process becomes easier. The best way of becoming aware of your extreme and unhelpful thinking is to try to notice times when your mood unhelpfully alters (e.g. at times when you feel upset) and then to ask 'What is going through my mind right now?'

The next section of this workbook will help you to move on to how to change these thoughts. Remember: we all have all sorts of thoughts during the day. The thoughts we need to focus on changing are those that are:

● **Extreme,** i.e. show one of the unhelpful thinking styles.
● **Unhelpful,** i.e. worsen how we feel and/or affect what we do.

Section 4 **Changing our extreme and unhelpful thoughts**

The following steps are a proven way of changing thoughts that are extreme and unhelpful. The first step is to disarm the thought. You can use as many or as few of the following steps as you need. Just stop when you feel you are able to move on from the thought.

The steps of the thought review are:

1 Label the thought as 'just one of those unhelpful thoughts'.
2 Stop, think and reflect: don't get caught up in it.
3 Move on, act against it, and don't be put off from what you were going to do.
4 Respond by giving yourself a truly compassionate response.

If you want to:

5 Act like a scientist: put the thought under a microscope and ask the seven thought-challenge questions.
6 Come to a balanced conclusion about what you've learned.
7 Experiment: test out what happens when you act on the balanced conclusion and against the extreme and unhelpful thought.

These steps are described below.

Step 1: label it as 'just one of those unhelpful thoughts'

All of us notice unhelpful thoughts from time to time. These thoughts can backfire and worsen how we feel. They are present more often at times when we are struggling.

 Choose a recent time when you have felt worse. Next, read through the list below and tick the unhelpful thinking patterns that were present at that time.

Unhelpful thinking style	Tick if your thought(s) showed this pattern at that time
Was I being my own worst critic? (bias against yourself)	
Was I focusing on the bad in situations? (negative mental filter)	
Was I making negative predictions about the future? (gloomy view of the future)	
Was I jumping to the very worst conclusion? (catastrophising)	
Was I second-guessing that others see me badly without checking whether this is actually true? (mind-reading)	
Was I taking unfair responsibility for things that aren't really my fault or taking all the blame?	
Was I using unhelpful 'must'/'should'/'ought'/'got to' statements? (making extreme statements or setting impossible standards)	

CHOICE POINT

If the thought doesn't show one of the unhelpful thinking styles, then you should stop here. Think about whether there were any other thoughts you noticed at the same time. Did any of them show an unhelpful thinking style? If so, they would be a better choice as an upsetting thought to change.

Step 2: stop, think and reflect: don't get caught up in it

Simply **noticing** that this is an unhelpful thinking style can be a powerful way of defusing it.

- **Label the upsetting thought as 'just another of those unhelpful/silly thoughts'.** These are just a part of what happens when we are upset. The thought will go away and lose its power. It's part of distress, not the true picture. Maybe say to the thought 'I've found you out – I'm not going to play that game again!'
- **Allow the thought to 'just be'.** Don't allow yourself to get caught up in it. Don't bother trying to challenge the thought or argue yourself out of it. Like a celebrity, such thoughts love attention. They're just not worth your attention. Allow them to **just be**. Take a mental step back from the thought as if observing it from a distance. Move your mind on to other, more helpful things, such as the future or recent achievements. Even better, move your mind on to the task in hand.

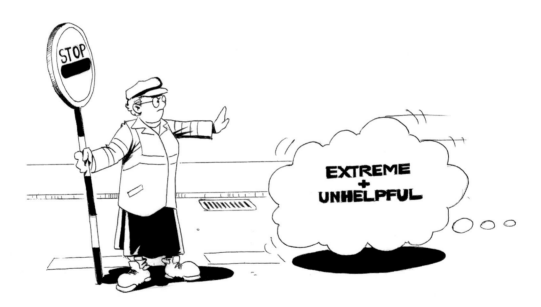

Step 3: move on, act against it, and don't be put off from what you were going to do

Unhelpful thinking worsens how you feel and unhelpfully alters what you do. The thought may cause you to:

- Stop, reduce or avoid doing something you were going to do. This leads to a loss of pleasure and achievement and, in the longer term, will restrict your life and undermine your confidence.
- Feel you must do something that is actually unhelpful, such as drinking too much alcohol. This ends up backfiring and worsening how you or others feel.

Make an **active choice** not to allow this to happen again. This often means acting against the thought. Choose to react helpfully rather than unhelpfully.

The big bully[1]

Extreme and unhelpful thoughts can enslave us. There is a compulsive aspect to them. Once we start worrying needlessly or become very negative, it is possible to get pushed about by our negative and fearful thoughts. Stopping, thinking and reflecting can help us avoid this pitfall.

Imagine a child who is bullied at school. We can understand how scared they may become and how they may hand over whatever the bully demands because they are terrified of being hurt or humiliated. In fact, this is quite a good short-term way of solving the problem. The child hands over their pocket money and the bully goes away. However, giving in to the bully makes it more likely that the bully will come back. In fact, the more the child gives, the more the bully returns. What would happen if, every time the bully returned, the child did not hand over what the bully wanted? It is easy to imagine the initial anxiety the child would feel, but bullies usually make empty threats. They also stop coming back if it is no longer worthwhile for them to do so. We can see the same pattern when we get caught up in going over thoughts again and again. Letting ourselves be pushed around by our thoughts actually doesn't help.

To stand up to the bully, try these three dos and three don'ts:

Three dos

- Keep doing what you planned to do anyway. Keep to your plan. Stay active.
- **Face your fears:** act against thoughts that tell you that things are too scary and you should avoid things. By creating a step-by-step approach, you can overcome these fears. See the workbook *Overcoming reduced activity and avoidance*.
- **Experiment:** if a thought says don't do something, do it! If a thought says you won't enjoy going to that wedding, try going and see whether you do enjoy it. You will find out more about this shortly.

Three don'ts

- Don't get pushed into not doing things by the thoughts.
- Don't live your life based on fear.
- Don't block how you feel by drinking alcohol or by using safety behaviours such as reassurance-seeking.

Why reassurance-seeking can be a problem

Reassurance-seeking can be quite subtle. None of us likes to admit we sometimes seek reassurance. But reassurance-seeking is a very human thing that we all do from time to time. This doesn't just mean seeking praise or approval from others. It also includes times when we feel anxious and look to others to reassure us that everything will be OK. Doing this from time to time isn't a problem. Sometimes, however, we can become dependent on needing this sort of reassurance. It then becomes a problem and ends up undermining how we feel and reducing our confidence. We end up feeling that we cannot do things without others. You can find out more about this in the workbook *Overcoming reduced activity and avoidance*.

Many people find that these few simple steps make a big difference. If you find you are still troubled by the thought, you may find these additional changes helpful. Again, try as many or as few of them as you feel you need.

---

[1] Thank you to Dale Huey for this example.

Step 4. Respond by giving yourself a truly compassionate response[2]

If a friend was troubled by a thought or worry, you would offer words of advice to soothe and encourage them. Imagine you have the best friend in the world – someone who is totally on your side, totally loving and totally compassionate. What words of advice and encouragement would they say to you?

Write their compassionate advice here:

....

....

....

Dwell on this: choose to apply their words in your own situation. Trust what they say. Allow that trust to wash over you and take away the troubling thoughts. Don't just view these as words; instead, try to get the right tone of warmth and compassion as you say the words to yourself.

You might choose a close friend, a relative, a famous person from literature or God. Whoever you choose, you need to be aware that the response will be unconditionally positive, compassionate and supportive.

(e.g.) EXAMPLE

Anne chooses her grandmother. She thinks back to what she would have said. These are words of support and love: 'You know we all love you, Anne. People often feel embarrassed when they feel ill – and Mary did come by without letting you know. Don't you worry about what you said to her. Anyone could have said that – it's not worth upsetting yourself about. You can always ask her round for coffee at a time that you decide. She'd love to come – you won't have put her off. Mary loves you too. She doesn't want to pressurise you – she just wants to help. And why don't you ask her to give you a ring before she pops by for the time being.'

 CHOICE POINT

Many people find that these four steps are enough to help change upsetting thoughts. They help you break the upsetting pattern of how you respond. If you find that after practising this approach on a number of thoughts over a week or so this is enough, then skip to Section 6. If you find that you need some more help with changing your thoughts, move on the next section.

---

[2]The concept of the 'compassionate mind' response was developed by Professor Paul Gilbert and is mentioned with his permission.

Section 5   **Challenging your thoughts**

Step 5: Act like a scientist: put the thought under a microscope and ask the seven thought-challenge questions

Our extreme and unhelpful thoughts are often inaccurate and untrue. Pretend you are a scientist approaching the issue in a completely logical way.

   Write down your thought on the space on the microscope slide below.

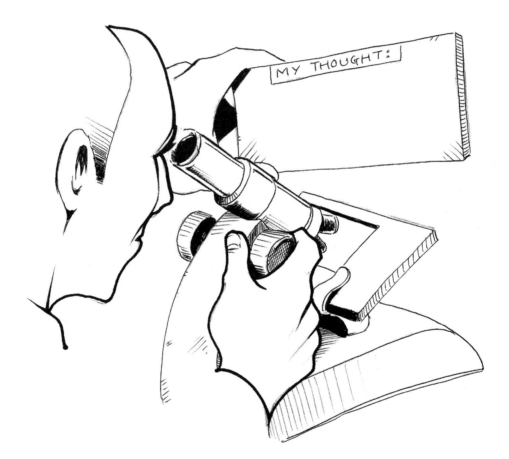

 First, rate **how much** you believe the upsetting thought. Make a cross on the line below to show how much you believed the thought at the time:

Not at all	Completely
0%	100%

It's easy to believe the worst when we are upset.

EXAMPLE

Paul's painting

Paul has very high standards and is currently feeling depressed and anxious. He has decided to paint his bedroom as a way of increasing his activity levels. He has just completed painting the walls when he realises that a drop of paint has fallen on to the carpet. He immediately feels down and angry with himself and thinks 'I always mess things up.' He rates his belief in this as 75% at the time.

Paul recognises that the thought shows one of the unhelpful thinking styles and is unhelpful. He tries to stop, think and reflect on it, and say something truly compassionate to himself. In spite of this, he feels upset, stops painting and goes to bed. Later on, he reflects that this upsetting thought would be a good one to challenge.

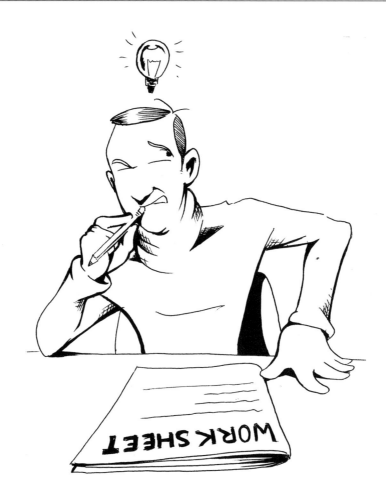

Answer the following questions, looking at Paul's example that follows if you need some hints and tips.

First, question the thought – don't just accept it. Is there **anything** to make you think the upsetting thought is incorrect? You might find it helpful to imagine you are in a court room demanding answers of the thought.

✎

....

....

....

EXAMPLE

'I had been painting for hours and was tired. I had put down dustsheets and they caught most of the drips. The rest of the painting went well. I even saw the drip so that I could clean it up and avoiding trampling it all over the house. I can't be expected to get everything right. It's silly to say "I always mess things up" – it was just one drip.'

The following seven questions will help you to **stop, think and reflect** to see whether there are any other things you need to bear in mind when answering this question. These questions are particularly effective at helping you to get a different perspective. Remember not to get caught up in the thought. Try to be completely objective.

Not every question will help you every time. Try them out. **Slow down** your reactions so you can really reflect on your answers.

? What would you tell a friend who said the same thing?

....

....

....

e.g. EXAMPLE

'I'd tell them "What are you saying? You're just being silly. The rest of the painting went well and the room looks great. Stop criticising yourself like that. You're just focusing on the drop of paint rather than the whole picture. You managed to use turps to remove most of the mark and it hasn't spoiled the floor. You don't *always* mess everything up." I'd also say, "Look at all the other things you have done this week. Give yourself due credit."'

? Are you basing this on how you feel rather than on the facts?

....

....

....

e.g. EXAMPLE

'It must be how I feel. Normally I would have just tried to clean up the drip or move some furniture to cover it up. I would have said "So what?" and got on with things. My mood must be affecting how I feel.'

(?) What would other people say?

✎

....

....

....

(e.g.) EXAMPLE

'Other people have said it looks good. My friend Alison liked it, and I trust her to say what she really thinks. Maybe I am wrong to say "I always mess things up". Alison doesn't think that.'

(?) Are you looking at the whole picture?

✎

....

....

....

(e.g.) EXAMPLE

'I actually did a good job. I prepared for it well, and the end job looks good. I should give myself credit for the positive job I did rather than focusing on one small thing that went wrong.'

(?) Does it **really** matter so much?

✎

....

....

....

(e.g.) EXAMPLE

'On a global scale of things, I guess not. It is just the painting. At least I've got somewhere to paint!'

(?) What would you say about this looking back in six months' time?

✎

....

....

....

EXAMPLE

'I'm pretty certain I will have forgotten it!'

? Do you apply one set of standards to yourself and another set of standards to others?

....

....

....

EXAMPLE

'Definitely! I've always been like that.'

Once you have completed this, look back on your answers and see whether you can summarise all the things you have considered as a balanced conclusion. This should be based on all your responses.

My balanced conclusion:

....

....

....

EXAMPLE

'The painting didn't go completely right, but I've managed to clean up the small spot of paint that I dropped. There is a mark there, but it's hardly noticeable. The rest of the room looks good and I'm a good painter. I have also got some other things right this week. I need to be less harsh on myself.'

Now, re-rate your belief in the upsetting thought:

Not at all	Completely
0%	100%

Now, rate your belief in the new balanced conclusion:

Not at all	Completely
0%	100%

EXAMPLE

Paul re-rates his thoughts. He believes the original upsetting thought only 25% now. Previously, he had believed it 75%. At the same time, he believes his new balanced conclusion about 90%. He has successfully been able to challenge the upsetting thought.

Step 6: experiment your way free from the thoughts

One powerful action to test the helpfulness and accuracy of the balanced conclusion is to act on the balanced conclusion believing it to be true, and to see what happens. This may mean choosing to **do the reverse** of what the upsetting thought may be telling you to do.

 EXAMPLE

You are asked to a party. Your initial reaction is to say no because you predict 'I won't enjoy it.' Try to **act against** this thought by going to the party in order to test out whether it is true. You may well find that the party goes better than you predicted and that you do enjoy it, at least a little. Think back to times in the past where things have happened that you were dreading but that turned out far better than you anticipated.

 IMPORTANT POINT

By far the best evidence for or against a thought can be found by looking at the consequences of what happens when you choose to act or not act on the thought. You can see some more examples below. **Reinforce** your balanced conclusions by acting on them. **Undermine** your extreme and unhelpful thoughts by acting against them.

Imagine yourself wearing the white lab coat of the scientist as you do this.

What the extreme and unhelpful thought tells you	Possible balanced conclusion	Possible experiment to test this out
1 Don't do something, e.g. you're invited to a party and your first reaction is 'Don't go to the party – you won't enjoy it'	'I might not enjoy it, but it might be more fun than I think. I often predict that I won't enjoy things and things work out better than I predict. I need to test this out by acting against it and going to the party'	**Test out the extreme and unhelpful thought by acting against it:** go to the party, and be aware of a tendency to withdraw from things – perhaps sitting in the corner and not talking to anyone. Choose to go, and choose to have a chat and a dance. This doesn't mean overcompensating and trying to be the life and soul – but do go. You may have a surprisingly good time

What the extreme and unhelpful thought tells you	Possible balanced conclusion	Possible experiment to test this out
2 They don't like me, e.g. you are in a canteen and see some people you know a little but not well. The thought 'They don't like me' pops into your head. This might lead you to sit somewhere away from them and pretend you didn't see them	'Maybe they don't like me – not everyone has to. But they've never been nasty to me before. They may like me or at least think I'm OK. It could well be I'm just mind-reading because I've low confidence at the moment. I need to test out this balanced conclusion by seeing how they react when I do talk to them'	**Test out the balanced conclusion:** choose to go up to them and ask whether you can join them. Smile and see how they respond. If the table is full, say hello and ask how they are. Then find your own table. NB: When planning experiments, it's important to predict what might happen if they say no. For example, if they are sitting there to have a meeting or for someone's birthday celebration, then it might not be appropriate to join them. If they say no, there may be reasons other than them not liking you
3 It will go horribly wrong and I'll mess it up, e.g. you are asked to give a short speech at a wedding. You have given speeches before. You've never liked it but you have coped before. Here, you immediately predict it will go horribly wrong. You may be tempted to say no and avoid it	'I'm not great at doing speeches, but it is important and it will mean a lot to them. I might not be a professional speaker but I can probably do it OK with practice. I might tell them I'll give it a go but I'll keep it short'	**Test out the extreme and unhelpful thought by acting against it:** say yes, and try to do something short. Prepare what you will say. Write it down and use cards to remind yourself. Practise the speech with a friend or a few friends. Visit the venue beforehand to get a feeling of the size of the place. Build up to what you do. On the day, try some anxiety-control techniques such as looking in turn at a few people who you know and who are sitting near you. Address your short talk to them. Other people may be there, but imagining you are chatting directly to one person may help. Again, you may be surprised and find out what a sense of achievement it is doing something that you fear
		NB: You need to be **realistic**. If you do this, it needs to be only 'good enough'. Go into it with an expectation that you'll be happy if it's OK. It doesn't need to be the best speech of the event. Shorter is usually better on such occasions

What the extreme and unhelpful thought tells you	Possible balanced conclusion	Possible experiment to test this out
		If you are extremely shy in public settings and have no previous similar experiences, it would be entirely sensible to say no and not choose this experiment. It would be **too big a first step**
4 You won't be able to cope. You have bad panic attacks in super-markets (just like Harvinder), e.g. you wake up on 1 January and think 'I'm going to beat this!' You promise yourself that as a first step, you will go to the busiest supermarket at the busiest time	That isn't a sensible thing to do. A better way would be to build up slowly to this, e.g. 'If I go to a smaller shop and slow down my shopping so I face my fears there, I'm more likely to succeed'	**Test out the balanced conclusion:** the most important things is to face fears in a step-by-step way. A very important thing to planning experiments is to **pace things**. Don't suddenly decide to go to the largest supermarket at the busiest time. Instead, make changes in a planned way. See the workbook *Overcoming reduced activity and avoidance*

One of the things about experiments is to pick experiments that you can do **now**. Don't be too ambitious. For example, sometimes people are extremely scared of public speaking or have panic attacks (like Harvinder) in specific situations. You cannot expect to suddenly jump to the scariest and most challenging situation.

Remember that to test it out, you need to do something that is:

- Realistic.
- Achievable.
- At the right **pace**. Don't bite off more than you can chew. You may need to work up to things one step at a time. See the workbook *Overcoming reduced activity and avoidance* for more detail on how to do this.

My plan for putting my balanced conclusion into practice

To act against the upsetting thought (e.g. examples 1 and 3 in the table above):

✎

....

....

....

To reinforce my new balanced conclusion (e.g. examples 2 and 4 in the table above):

✎

....

....

....

Have you created a **plan** to put your balanced conclusion into practice?   Yes ☐   No ☐

---

e.g. **EXAMPLE**

Paul's plan for putting his balanced conclusion into practice

1 'I am going to choose to have a more helpful focus for my thinking. I'm going to set aside some time to think back on those things where I have a sense of achievement. I am going to choose to look at the whole room that I've painted, and not unhelpfully focus on the small spot of paint that is hardly noticeable. This will act against my tendency to focus on my failures.'

2 'I am going to choose to keep doing the painting and I am going to do this at a sensible pace. I will do the skirting boards tomorrow. That will help me to undermine that old thought that I always mess things up, because it will mean me acting against my tendency to go to bed and stop doing things. Sure, some things won't go completely right, but lots of things will go well, and it will be a lot more helpful for me to focus on these. Anyway, who does get everything right?'

3 'I'm going to ask my other friends what they think of the room and see whether they mention the spot of paint on the carpet. Now I come to think of it, I bet they don't.' (In fact, when he asks two other friends, they don't mention it at all. They do, however, say how impressed they are with the room.)

Think about your own experiment. Before you do this, write down exactly what you predict will happen. Rate any anxiety and fear, and then do it anyway.

Write down any extreme and unhelpful thoughts you notice. Record how much you believe them at the time, from 0% (not at all) to 100% (fully).

My thought(s):

....

....

....

I believed this   % **before** the experiment.

I believed this   % **during** the experiment.

I believed this   % **after** the experiment.

My level of anxiety:

% **before** the experiment.

% **during** the experiment.

% **after** the experiment.

Review the outcome

Write what happened here:

✎

....

....

....

(?) Was the experiment helpful?   Yes ☐   No ☐

(?) Did it help me to test out my fears and balanced conclusion?   Yes ☐   No ☐

(?) Overall, what have I learned from what happened about myself/others?

✎

....

....

....

(?) Overall, what have I learned from what happened about the original upsetting thought and about the balanced conclusion?

✎

....

....

....

Finally, come to an overall summary based on all the information you have about the unhelpful thought.

Workbook summary

In this workbook, you have:
- Learned how to notice patterns of extreme and unhelpful thinking that worsen how you feel.
- Discovered how to change extreme and unhelpful thinking.
- Learned how to experiment and test out your thinking.
- Discovered some ways of coming up with more balanced thoughts.
- Learned what to do if thoughts go round and round in your head.

The approach you have worked through can be applied to any unhelpful thoughts that result in you feeling worse. By labelling, stepping back from and occasionally challenging these thoughts, you will begin to change the way you see yourself, your current situation and the future.

Putting into practice what you have learned

You will find blank thought practice worksheets at the end of this workbook. Copy them if you require further sheets. You can also download further sheets from www.livinglifetothefull.com.

Getting the most from the thought worksheets

To get the most from the worksheets:
- Practise using the approach whenever you notice your mood altering unhelpfully. With practice, you will find it easier to notice and change your own extreme and unhelpful thinking.
- Try to react to your unhelpful thoughts as soon as possible after you notice your mood changing.
- If you cannot do this immediately, try to think yourself back into the situation so that you are as clear as possible in your answers later on when you do this task.
- With practice, you will find that you can take the most effective aspects of the sheets and use what works for you in everyday life.

Acknowledgements

I wish to thank all those who have commented upon this workbook, especially Theresa O'Brien, Marie Chellingsworth, Liz Rafferty, Ann McCreath and Susan Ross.

My notes

✎

....
....
....
....
....
....
....
....
....
....
....
....
....
....
....
....
....
....
....
....
....
....
....
....

My notes

✎

....

Practice sheets: my thought review of a time when I felt worse

Write in your experience in all five areas:

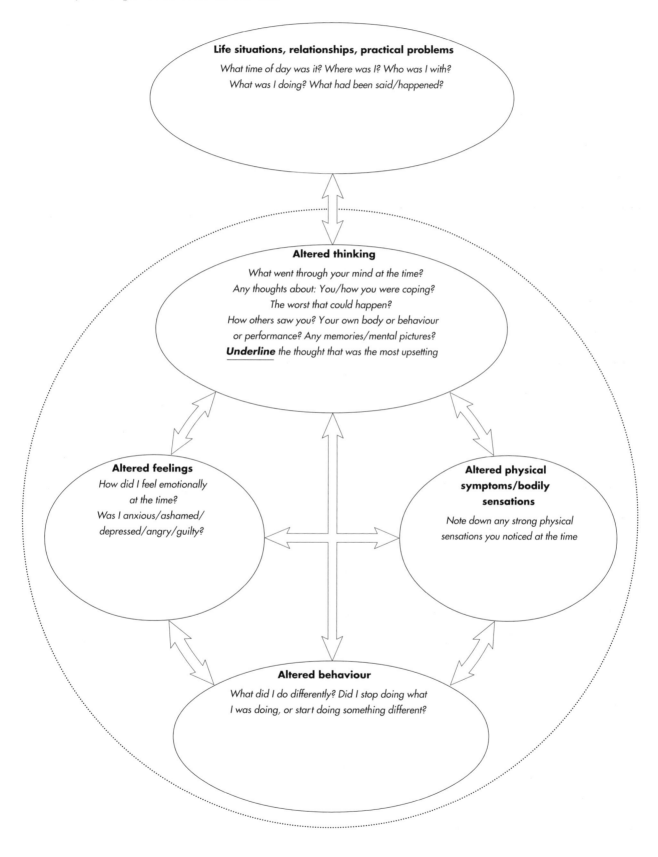

Life situations, relationships, practical problems

What time of day was it? Where was I? Who was I with?
What was I doing? What had been said/happened?

Altered thinking

What went through your mind at the time?
Any thoughts about: You/how you were coping?
The worst that could happen?
How others saw you? Your own body or behaviour
or performance? Any memories/mental pictures?
***Underline** the thought that was the most upsetting*

Altered feelings

How did I feel emotionally
at the time?
Was I anxious/ashamed/
depressed/angry/guilty?

Altered physical
symptoms/bodily
sensations

Note down any strong physical
sensations you noticed at the time

Altered behaviour

What did I do differently? Did I stop doing what
I was doing, or start doing something different?

Summary

The key steps of the thought review are:

- **Label it** as 'just one of those unhelpful thoughts'.
  - Am I being my own worst critic? (Bias against yourself.)
  - Am I focusing on the bad in situations? (Negative mental filter.)
  - Am I making negative predictions about the future? (Gloomy view of the future.)
  - Am I jumping to the very worst conclusion? (Catastrophising.)
  - Am I second-guessing that others see me badly without actually checking whether this is actually true? (Mind-reading.)
  - Am I taking unfair responsibility for things that aren't really my fault or taking all the blame?
  - Am I using unhelpful 'must'/'should'/'ought'/'got to' statements? (Making extreme statements or setting impossible standards.)
- **Stop think and reflect:** don't get caught up in it.
- **Move on:** don't be put off from what you were going to do. Keep active. Face your fears. Keep to your plan. Respond helpfully.
- Give yourself a **truly compassionate response**, e.g. what would someone who loved you really say?

If you want to:

- **Act like a scientist:** put the thought under a microscope. Ask the seven thought-challenge questions. First, rate how much you believe the thought (0–100%). Then ask:
  - What would I tell a friend who said the same thing?
  - Am I basing this on how I feel rather than the facts?
  - What would other people say?
  - Am I looking at the whole picture?
  - Does it really matter so much?
  - What would I say about this, looking back in six months' time?
  - Do I apply one set of standards to myself and another set to others?
- **Experiment:** test it out and come to a balanced conclusion. Act against the original extreme thought. Act on your new balanced conclusion – see what happens.
- Finally, come to a **summary** based on everything you have learned.

Re-rate how much you believe the original upsetting thought (0–100%) and the new balanced conclusion.

Remember: this process takes time. With practice, you will build your confidence in using the approach.

 A credit-card-sized version of this is available free of charge from www.livinglifetothefull.com. Printed versions are also available to order. Larger worksheets to identify and challenge extreme and unhelpful thoughts are also available.

Overcoming reduced activity and avoidance

Dr Chris Williams

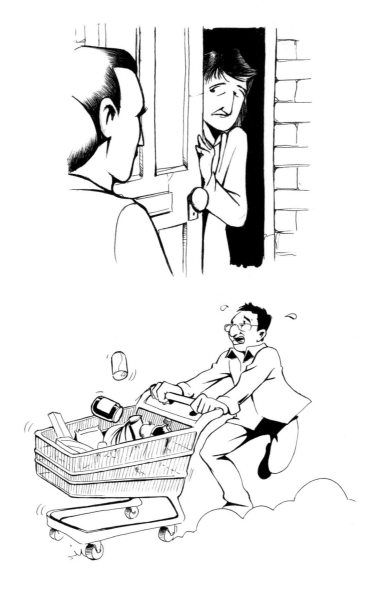

A Five Areas Approach
Helping you to help yourself
www.livinglifetothefull.com

Section 1   Introduction

Symptoms of all sorts can affect our activity levels and restrict what we are able to do.

In this workbook you will:

- Discover how symptoms affect our lives.
- Identify any reduced activity and avoidance in your own life and consider the impact on you.
- Learn how to record your current activity levels.
- See examples of ways of overcoming reduced activity and avoidance.
- Practise this approach yourself in order to make slow, steady changes to your life.
- Plan some next steps to build on this improvement.

The impact of symptoms on our lives

The experience of feeling unwell affects everyone in unique ways. At the same time, how we respond tends to fall into one of several common patterns of responding. This workbook focuses on helping you identify patterns of reduced activity and avoidance.

The impact of reduced activity

When you notice symptoms, it is normal to find it difficult to do things. This may be because of:

- Low energy and tiredness ('I'm too tired').
- Low mood and little sense of enjoyment or achievement when things are done.
- Symptoms getting in the way, e.g. pain, weakness or restricted movement, which can make getting out difficult.
- Negative thinking and reduced enthusiasm to do things ('I just can't be bothered').

The result is reduced activity. Although this is understandable, it can make us feel even worse. We can become so preoccupied that other important things in life are squeezed out. We focus instead on core life activities that we **have** to do. This might include the mechanics of looking after children, doing chores or just struggling to get by. Other things that we would usually do for fun can slowly just drop away.

For example, we may cut down on doing hobbies, talking with family, going out for walks, reading books or magazines for fun, meeting up with friends, or listening to music. We may become so focused on just surviving that we don't have time to sit back and feel a sense of achievement in what we do.

The result is:

- **We feel lower in mood:** we have emptied our lives of the things that give us a sense of pleasure and achievement. We also lose our feelings of **closeness** to other people and stop doing things we really value.
- **We feel physically worse:** if there is a very large reduction in activity levels, this may lead to problems of weakness, stiffness and pain in underused muscles and joints.

Sometimes, we can feel as though everything is just too much effort. A pattern of reduced activity may result. This is sometimes called a **vicious circle of reduced activity**. The responses add to our problems and worsen how we feel.

The consequences of inactivity

When we feel ill, a natural response is to rest in order to allow recovery. Resting can be helpful sometimes – for example, to allow acute inflammation to settle. However, there may also be unintended consequences.

For example, unused muscles tend to lose muscle bulk and weaken. A research study investigated students who were paid to go to bed for several months. The study showed that the students lost about 10% of their muscle bulk and strength in the first week of bed rest and a further 10% over subsequent weeks. The lesson learned from this is that resting can worsen symptoms.

Rest can also create muscle and joint pain. When we rest excessively, we tend to stiffen up. This is especially true when we lie down or sit in a chair for hours on end. Often, a slow steady increase in activity can help. This helps improves our mobility and reduces pain. For this reason, physiotherapists and doctors advise people to try to maintain activity levels as much as possible.

 EXAMPLE

Anne is living with problems of low back pain. The months of pain have made it difficult for her to get out, and she is no longer able to get in to work. She has been off work now for 14 months. In spite of her health problems, she has coped remarkably well. She lives in a ground-floor flat overlooking the local park. Before she was ill, she used to enjoy walking across to the park and chatting to people cycling, walking and playing football there. She loves listening to music and talk shows on the radio and also reading. She has a small circle of good friends she met through work, and she keeps in close contact with her brother and sister. She is especially fond of her brother's children – her nephew Tom and her niece Sarah – who she used to see very often.

However, her brother and his family moved away at the start of the year. Although they talk by phone, it isn't the same. For the past six months, Anne has really struggled with worsening pain and also feeling increasingly low and upset. She has become more and more isolated and sits crying, looking at photos of the family. She is doing far less than usual. She hasn't told her brother anything, and she puts on a brave face. She has stopped reading, and now the radio is left switched off. She no longer walks to the park, but instead sits alone in her chair. When she thinks of her situation, she sees herself as a failure and believes she will never get back to work. Physically she feels stiffer and stiffer. She finds she can only walk for a few minutes without having to stop and rest.

---

task Write Anne's symptoms into the figure below to summarise her vicious circle of reduced activity.

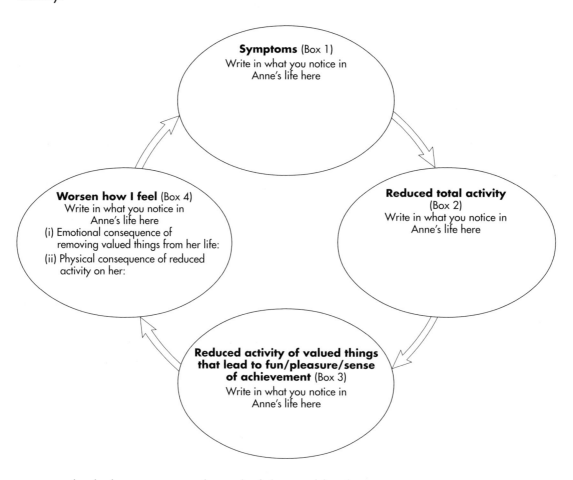

Hint: you can check the answers at the end of the workbook.

? Does a similar pattern of reduced activity apply to you? Are there any things you have reduced or stopped doing since you started to feel like you do? Write them into the box below.

....

....

....

? With reference to the vicious circle in the figure above, answer the following questions:

Have I stopped doing things I used to enjoy as a result of how I feel?	Yes ☐	No ☐	Sometimes ☐
Has the reduced activity removed things from life that previously gave me a sense of pleasure or achievement?	Yes ☐	No ☐	Sometimes ☐
Has the reduced activity worsened how I feel emotionally or physically?	Yes ☐	No ☐	Sometimes ☐
Overall, has this worsened how I feel?	Yes ☐	No ☐	Sometimes ☐

If you have answered yes or sometimes to all four questions, then you are experiencing a vicious circle of reduced activity. The good news is that if you are experiencing this, then this is something you can plan to change, as described in Section 3 later.

The impact of avoidance

When somebody develops symptoms, they often become worried about what they can and can't do. Sometimes these concerns cause them to avoid things such as:

- **Going to particular places or getting into situations** where they predict they will feel worse. For example, people who fear feeling worse in shops because of panic (sometimes called agoraphobia) will avoid going into larger, busier shops. Similarly, someone who experiences high levels of anxiety in social settings will try very hard to avoid such situations.

- **Activities they fear might make them worse, such as physical exercise or sex.** Sometimes we can become concerned about the impact physical activity may have upon us. We may be concerned about overdoing things that might feel too much. This avoidance is entirely appropriate if there is a clear physical reason to limit things, for example if there is heart disease that causes severe angina. However, sometimes our avoidance can become excessive and inappropriate. For example, someone with exercise-induced asthma may become so anxious about causing another attack that they avoid **any** hint of activity. They lose confidence in their ability to do any strenuous activity 'just in case' it makes them worse. This avoidance flies in the face of medical advice to maintain a healthy lifestyle. Similarly, a person with angina might completely avoid sex. This is in spite of the fact that, medically, there is no reason why sex cannot be enjoyed in the vast majority of cases. Here, the fear is of getting so excited or exerted that a heart attack may occur.

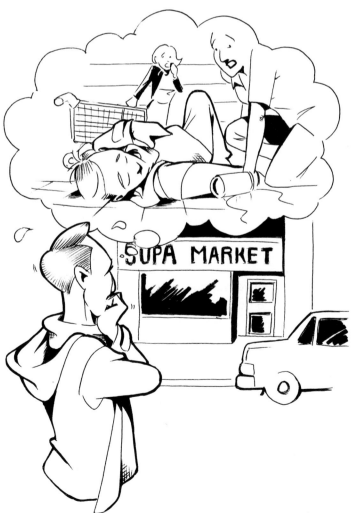

This avoidance adds to the person's problems. A pattern of worsening avoidance often results. This is sometimes called a **vicious circle of avoidance**.

 Write here any examples of avoidance you have noticed:

✎

....

....

....

The problem with avoidance is that it teaches us the unhelpful rule that the **only** way to deal with a difficult situation is through avoiding it. In fact, often the most effective way of tackling our fears is to face up to them in a planned, step-by-step way. The avoidance also reduces the opportunities we have to test out whether our fears are actually true. It therefore worsens anxiety and undermines our confidence even further. This process is summarised in the diagram below.

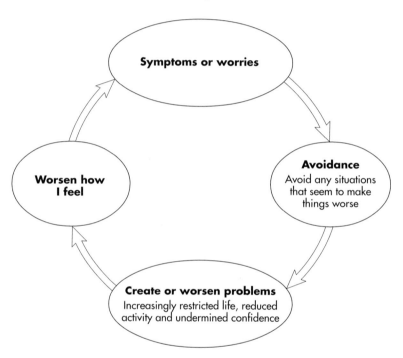

(e.g.) EXAMPLE

Harvinder has panic attacks whenever he goes to a supermarket. He says 'I'm not going to large shops at all now because I'd get panicky. I'd feel really hot and sweaty and start breathing very fast. I'd be scared I'd collapse. Instead, I'll go to the small local shops at the quietest possible time. I always choose the shortest queue because of anxiety rather than because it is the obvious choice.'

Look at the circle above. Because of his panic symptoms, Harvinder is avoiding things. This is undermining his confidence and adding to his problems.

To see whether this pattern applies to you, ask yourself 'What have I stopped or avoided doing because of my worries or concerns?' Remember that, at times, the avoidance can be quite **subtle**, for example choosing to go to the shops at a time when you know they are quiet and then rushing through the shopping as quickly as possible.

Having completed these questions, reflect on your answers using the three questions below:

Am I avoiding things or doing certain actions that are designed to improve how I feel?	Yes ☐	No ☐	Sometimes ☐
Has this reduced my confidence in things and led to an increasingly restricted life?	Yes ☐	No ☐	Sometimes ☐
Overall, has this worsened how I feel?	Yes ☐	No ☐	Sometimes ☐

If you have answered yes or sometimes to all three questions, then you are experiencing a vicious circle of avoidance.

The good news is that once you have noticed whether avoidance or reduced activity are occurring in your own life, then you can start to tackle this in a planned, step-by-step way. You will find out how to do this in the next section of this workbook.

Section 2 First steps to tackling reduced activity and avoidance

We may have made all sorts of previous attempts to change but, unless we have a clear plan and stick to it, change will be difficult. Selecting the changes to try first is the crucial first part of successfully moving forwards. By choosing the activities to focus on to start with, you are actively choosing at first **not** to focus on other areas.

Setting targets will help you to focus on how to make the changes needed in order to get better. To do this, you will need to decide:

- **Short-term targets:** thinking about changes you can make today, tomorrow and the next week.
- **Medium-term targets:** changes to be put in place over the next few weeks.
- **Long-term targets:** where you want to be in six months or a year.

Reviewing your activities

The first step to making changes is **recording** what you are currently able to do. An **activity diary** can help you summarise this and provides a baseline on which to build.

Rate **each** activity you do each day for:

- The **pleasure** experienced, on a scale of 0–10.
- How much of an **achievement** it was, on a scale of 0–10.

0	5	10
No pleasure or achievement	Feel OK/reasonable	Complete pleasure or achievement

NB: you need to answer these bearing in mind how much your symptoms are currently affecting your ability to do things. You need to be fair on yourself in how you judge this.

(e.g.) EXAMPLE

Someone is struggling to maintain the activities they did before. In spite of this, it is likely that some life activities will continue to provide a sense of pleasure and achievement. For example, going out for a walk may give a score of 6/10 for pleasure. It may also rate as 7/10 for achievement: they didn't want to go and they found it difficult, but they managed it anyway.

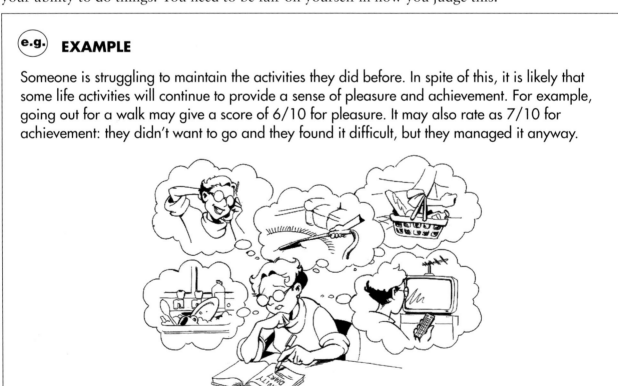

What activities should I record?

Use the **activity diary** at the end of this workbook to record **everything** that you do over the next few days. This might include:

- Getting dressed.
- Talking to a friend on the phone.
- Doing some housework.
- Going shopping.
- Washing your hair.
- Doing the washing up.

Include times when you are watching TV, having a bath, resting, etc.

An example of Anne's completed **activity diary** is given on page 10. This shows that even though Anne is doing less than usual (she's no longer going to the park), she is still doing some things. Importantly, a number of these activities are helping her feel better.

 IMPORTANT POINT

It is very important when completing the activity diary to watch out for negative thoughts that may cause you to overlook your achievements. For someone who is struggling to cope, the previously simple act of getting up and dressed can be a very large achievement. Symptoms such as lack of energy, pain and tiredness can interfere significantly with your ability to carry out activities that most people do automatically. It is easy when feeling like this to think 'Well, I should do that anyway – anyone could do that' and discount your achievements. Try to watch out for these negative thoughts and **write down what you did** anyway.

e.g. EXAMPLE

Anne's activity diary

Date and time	Activity (include everything you do)	Duration (how long did you do it for?)	Pleasure felt (0 = no pleasure; 10 = maximum pleasure)	Sense of achievement gained (0 = no sense of achievement; 10 = maximum sense of achievement)
6–7 a.m.	In bed, asleep	7 hours	–	–
7–8 a.m.	Woke up and listened to the radio	30 minutes	1	2
8–9 a.m.	Got up, had a shower and cleaned my teeth	40 minutes	3	6
9–10 a.m.	Made coffee	15 minutes	5	5
10–11 a.m.	Watched television	90 minutes	4	2
11–12 p.m.	Watched television	50 minutes	5	2
12–1 p.m.	Friend called by and made them a drink	45 minutes	7	8

0   5   10

No pleasure or achievement   Feel OK/reasonable   Complete pleasure or achievement

task Keep an activity diary yourself today and for the next few days. You will find an activity diary at the back of this workbook to tear out or copy. Don't forget to include what you're doing at the moment – reading this workbook! Alternatively, you can use a diary or blank piece of paper. Write down what you do throughout the day. Use it to identify **patterns** in what you do and don't do. You will use it to help you to work out a first target to change in the next section of the workbook.

The purpose of doing this is to allow you to gather information to help you understand how your symptoms affect you. This will help you to plan specific changes to your life. Most people need to practise gathering this information for at least a few days in order to begin to work out the relationship between their activity and how they feel.

The activity diary will give you an idea of what sorts of things you have reduced or avoided doing. The aim is to help you discover whether any activities or situations are linked specifically to you feeling better or worse.

Taking enjoyment from your achievements

 task Use your activity diary to record positive events such as conversations and activities that gave you a sense of pleasure or achievement. Think back on the areas in the week that have been pleasurable. Use this approach to try to develop a more helpful focus to your thinking. Build in a time each day to reflect on these events and remember them. Choose to focus on and remember positive things.

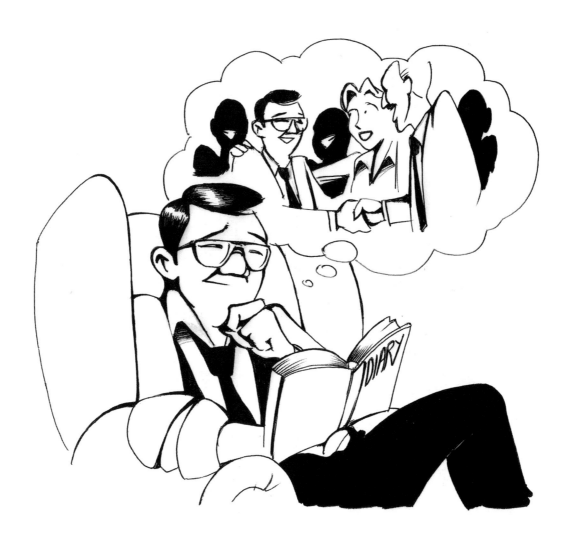

This idea of choosing to build in a helpful focus to at least part of your day can help boost your mood. Try this approach to see whether it is helpful for you.

How the activity diary can help you move forwards

Sometimes, it can be tempting to introduce changes into your life too quickly. If you find that you have got into a habit of doing very little and then suddenly throw yourself into doing too much, things can backfire. **Overdoing things can sometimes be just as unhelpful as underdoing things.** This so-called **all-or-nothing** response is shown by the solid line on the graph below. Here, the person throws themselves into things on days when they feel better. The problem is that they then crash back. The result is that, on average, they do less and less – as shown by the dotted line in the graph.

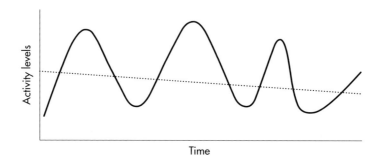

For example, if you feel good one day, do you tend to try to accomplish many things, leaving you exhausted for the next few days? This can also happen when you have a good week and feel almost back to your usual self. This **all-or-nothing cycle** is most common when you feel at your worst but also when you are recovering. It can be very frustrating and make it difficult to plan your life.

Say you are cutting the grass. A paced approach would include taking a break halfway through. In contrast, an all-or-nothing approach would mean throwing yourself into cutting the grass all at once and exhausting yourself in the process, as illustrated below.

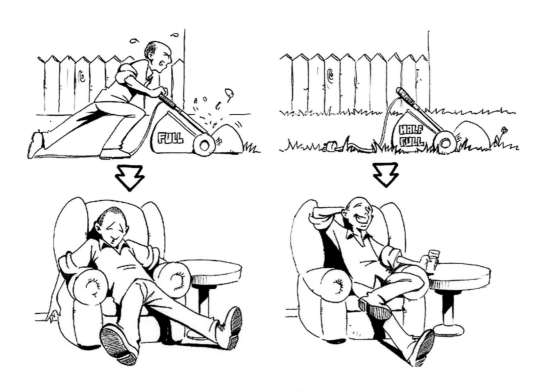

If this applies to you, the most crucial thing is to stabilise your activity and then build things up from there. Use the activity diary for a few days to start with. Often, it is easier to do this as you go along rather than trying to remember to fill it in at the end of the day. It will give you an idea of whether you are in an all-or-nothing cycle. Some people are surprised to find patterns emerging in what they do and how it makes them feel.

Once you have an idea of your current activity level, you can then build on this to pace yourself and increase your activity levels. You can plan this using the same diary sheet but this time completing it in advance with a plan of what you will do. For many people, this means that at first they might actually **reduce** what they are currently doing. The best way of using the diary sheet is to write a plan that is balanced and reasonable – and then stick to it. This can feel very unnatural at first. For example, some days you may be able to do all of the washing and most of the ironing. Other days, you may find it really hard to get up and do any laundry at all. A better situation would therefore be to be able to do some laundry every day. In this way, the all-or-nothing pattern can be broken. This way of changing your behaviour is known as **pacing**.

Another example is poor concentration stopping you finishing a crossword or sudoku puzzle or reading your newspaper. Again, finishing the crossword might seem easy sometimes but impossible at other times. It might seem a little strange at first, but pacing can help with this too. Plan with the diary what you will do, and use this to stabilise and then slowly pace an increase in what you do.

You will find out how to plan pacing in your own life in the next section of this workbook.

Section *3* Overcoming reduced activity and avoidance

Overview: the seven-step plan

By working through the seven steps outlined below, you can learn an approach that will help you to plan clear ways of overcoming any problems of reduced activity or avoidance. The aim isn't to change things across the board. Instead, the aim is to slowly increase **specific** activities in order to boost your confidence and feelings of pleasure and achievement.

Step 1: identify and define the problem as precisely as possible

You will already have an idea of the different activities you are doing – and not doing – from your activity diary.

 The following table summarises activities that are commonly affected. A wide range of altered behaviours have been summarised here to help you think about the changes that may occur. It is likely that you will have noticed changes in at least some of these activities.

As a result of how I feel, am I:	Tick here if you have noticed this, even if only sometimes
Stopping or reducing doing hobbies or interests, such as reading, or other things I previously enjoyed or did to relax?	
Going out or socialising less?	
Eating poorly, e.g. eating less or tending to eat more junk food or food that takes little preparation?	
Noticing physical consequences of reduced activity, e.g. worsened stiffness or pain, restricted joint movement or slowly worsening weakness of underused muscles?	
Brooding over things and therefore no longer living life to the full?	
Failing to keep up with housework, e.g. 'letting things go' around the house?	
Not always answering the phone or the door when people visit?	
Leaving letters and bills unopened or not replying to them because of a lack of energy or interest in actively dealing with them?	
Paying less attention to my self-care or personal hygiene, e.g. washing less, being less bothered about my appearance, wearing clothes for longer before washing them, not shaving or combing my hair?	

As a result of how I feel, am I:	**Tick here if you have noticed this, even if only sometimes**

Less interested in sex, e.g. physically pushing my partner away because of a lack of enjoyment in or energy for sex?

Staying inactive or in bed, so that I am far less physically active than before?

If you have a faith: no longer reading the scriptures, praying or going to my place of worship? (Have you stopped letting God in on the small and big things in life?)

(?) Have I reduced or stopped doing any other things? Write them here:

....

....

....

(?)

As a result of feeling anxious or worried, am I:	**Tick here if you have noticed this, even if only sometimes**

Avoiding specific situations, objects, places or people because of fears about what harm might result?

Avoiding dealing with important practical problems (large and small)?

Not really being honest with others, e.g. saying yes when really I mean no or not saying things that I really want to?

Trying hard to avoid situations that bring about upsetting thoughts or memories?

Avoiding physical activity or exercise that I should be able to do, as a result of concerns about my physical health?

Avoiding opening or replying to letters or bills?

Sleeping in to avoid doing things or meeting people?

Looking to others to sort things out for us?

Avoiding answering the phone or the door when people visit?

Avoiding sex?

Avoiding talking to others face to face?

Avoiding being with others in crowded or hot places? Avoiding busy or large shops?

As a result of feeling anxious or worried, am I: **Tick here if you have noticed this, even if only sometimes**

Avoiding going on buses, in cars or any places from where it is difficult to
   escape?

Avoiding walking alone far from home?

No longer attending religious services, night classes or local pubs and
   clubs because it feels just too much to cope with at present?

(?) Am I avoiding things in other ways? Write here how you are doing this if this is applicable
   to you.

....

....

....

Look back at your list and from this identify a **single** initial target area that you will focus on.
This is particularly important if you have ticked a number of boxes in the checklist. It is not
possible to overcome all these areas at once. Instead, you need to choose **one** area on which to
focus to start with.

   My target area: write one problem area that you want to work on. Remember that this should
be a problem of reduced activity or avoidance that is worsening how you feel:

....

....

....

It may be that the thought of making changes here seems daunting or impossible. The key is to
use a **step-by-step** approach where no step seems too large. The first step needs to be something
that gets you moving in the right direction.

   Ask yourself whether you need to break down the problem area into a number of smaller, more
achievable targets. You can do this by funnelling down from a general area of reduced activity or
avoidance to a more specific target that you can tackle first.

(?) Is this a small, focused problem that is a realistic target for change
   over the next week or so?   Yes ☐   No ☐

CHOICE POINT

If you answer yes, skip to Step 2. If you answer no, keep reading about how to identify a
realistic first target.

Funnelling down: choosing a clear first step on which to work

What smaller steps do you need to tackle first? Select a smaller aspect of the problem that you wish to change at the present time. Write it here. This should be a problem of reduced activity or avoidance – not an issue to do with your own thoughts or emotions:

✎

....

....

....

(?)

Is this a clear, focused problem?	Yes ☐	No ☐
Is it realistic, practical and achievable?	Yes ☐	No ☐

If you answer no to either of these questions, rewrite your target problem here:

✎

....

....

....

Reality check: is this a realistic target for change? Imagine that throughout your entire life, you've never done any exercise. Then you decide to run the London Marathon as your first step. There is no way you can go from a situation of little exercise to suddenly running a marathon. We have to be realistic: any change we make needs to push us but should also be realistic and achievable. Going swimming is a better first target.

(e.g.) EXAMPLE

Anne's target of what she wants to change first

'I have stopped meeting up with lots of friends.'

(e.g.) EXAMPLE

Harvinder's target of what he wants to change first

'Tackling my avoidance of large and busy shops/supermarkets.'

It may be that the thought of making changes seems daunting or impossible. The key is to use a **step-by-step** approach where no step seems too large.

Step 2: think up as many solutions as possible in order to achieve your initial goal

The purpose of brainstorming is to come up with as many ideas as possible. Among them you hope to be able to identify a realistic, practical and achievable solution. Completely wacky ideas should be included as well, even if you would never choose them in practice. This can help you adopt a flexible approach to the problem.

Try to **think broadly**. Useful questions to help you to think up possible solutions might include:

- What advice would you give a friend who was trying to tackle the same problem? (Sometimes we can more easily think of solutions for others than for ourselves.)
- What ridiculous solutions can I include, as well as more sensible ideas?
- What helpful suggestions would others (e.g. family, friends and work colleagues) make?
- How could I look at the solutions facing me differently? For example, what would I have said before I felt like this, or what might I say about the situation in five years' time?
- What approaches have I tried in the past in similar circumstances?

If you feel stuck, sometimes doing this task with someone you trust can be helpful.

 EXAMPLE

Anne's ideas for tackling her reduced activity

Anne gets a piece of paper and writes down possible ways she could start to meet up with her friends again. She includes wacky ideas as well as more sensible ones. Here is Anne's list:

- Hire a hall and a band and invite all my friends to a party.
- Ask my friend Sarah round for coffee.
- Phone my friend Sarah.
- Have a meal out at a local restaurant with friends.
- Cook a meal at home and invite some friends.

 EXAMPLE

Harvinder's ideas for tackling his avoidance

- Contact the manager of a supermarket and pay them a lot of money to arrange a personal evening opening when I can shop alone.
- Go into the largest busiest shop I can find and stay there until I feel better.
- Take part in a sponsored shop for charity.
- Go to a local smaller shop but don't rush through the shopping.
- Go to the post office at the busiest time and join the longest queue.

Brainstorming my own problem

Write down as many possible options (including ridiculous ideas at first) to help you tackle your own problem:

✎

....

....

....

....

....

....

....

....

Step 3: look at the advantages and disadvantages of each possible solution

The next step is to think about the pros and cons of each possible option.

Below is Anne's list of advantages and disadvantages:

Suggestion	Advantages	Disadvantages
1 Hire a hall and a band and invite all my friends to a party	I'd meet lots of people; it might be fun	The idea is far too scary; I know I couldn't cope with it at the moment; anyway, it would cost a fortune and I can't afford that sort of thing
2 Ask my friend Sarah round for coffee	I like Sarah and it would be nice to catch up; she's been on holiday and I want to know whether she met anyone there	This is only a little bit scary, but how would the conversation go? There may be some long, embarrassing silences
3 Phone my friend Sarah	We always used to natter on the phone and we used to enjoy it; she's one of my oldest friends so it would probably be easy	I haven't spoken to her for at least two months and I'm not sure what we would talk about
4 Have a meal out with friends at a local restaurant	I like curry and it would give me a chance to catch up with my friends	Again, I'm not so sure about this. It feels like this might be going a step too far. It might feel like a very long night, and I'm not sure I can cope
5 Cook a meal at home and invite some friends	I like cooking and it would give a focus for me to work towards	It could go wrong; it would put me under a lot of pressure getting all the food in; I'm not sure how many people I should invite; this seems even more stressful

Harvinder uses a similar approach (not summarised here). Look back at his list and think for yourself about the pluses and minuses of each of his five possible targets.

My advantages and disadvantages

Next, write in the pros and cons for your own suggested first steps:

Suggestion	Advantages	Disadvantages

Step 4: choose one of the solutions

The chosen solution should be an option that will make a sensible first step in tackling your problem. It should be realistic and likely to succeed. The decision needs to be based on all your answers to Step 3.

In making your decision, it is important to bear in mind that the most effective ways of tackling avoidance and reduced activity are to plan a **steady, slow increase** in activity. By making step-by-step changes, you can slowly tackle your problems and rebuild your confidence. The sort of solution you are looking for is, therefore, something that gets you moving in the right direction. This should be small enough to be possible but big enough to move you forwards.

EXAMPLE

Anne's reduced activity

Anne decides on option 3 – 'Phone my friend Sarah'. Option 2 (to ask Sarah round for a coffee) might also have been possible, but on balance Anne prefers option 3, as it seemed to be more realistic, practical and achievable at present.

 EXAMPLE

Harvinder's avoidance

Harvinder decides to go to a local smaller shop but this time to not rush through his shopping.

KEY POINT

The first step should be something that helps you tackle your avoidance or reduced activity. If it seems scary, it should not be so scary that you can't do it. You must be realistic in your choice so that the target does not appear impossible.

Look at your own responses in Step 3. From this, you should choose a solution. Write your preferred solution here:

....

....

....

This solution should be an option that fulfils the following three criteria:

Is it **useful** for changing how you are?	Yes ☐	No ☐
Is it a **clear task**, so that you will know when you have done it?	Yes ☐	No ☐
Is it something that is realistic, practical and achievable?	Yes ☐	No ☐

Step 5: plan the steps needed to carry it out

 IMPORTANT POINT

You need to generate a clear plan that will help you to decide exactly **what** you are going to do and **when** you are going to do it. It is useful to **write down** the steps needed to carry out your solution. This helps you to plan what to do and allows you to predict possible problems that might arise. Remember to build into your plan some thought about what you will do if the plan doesn't succeed fully.

My plan to increase my activity levels

Write your plan down here. Include how you will tackle any possible blocks that might get in the way:

✎

....
....
....
....
....
....
....
....
....
....
....
....
....
....
....
....
....

Your task is to carry this out during the next week.

This is the key part of the problem-solving process. Be as precise as possible in your plan. Next, apply the questions for effective change to your plan in order to check how practical and achievable it is.

The questions for effective change

Is the planned activity one that:

Will be useful for understanding or changing how I am?	Yes ☐	No ☐
Is a specific task, so that I will know when I have done it?	Yes ☐	No ☐
Is realistic, practical and achievable?	Yes ☐	No ☐
Makes clear what I am going to do and when I am going to do it?	Yes ☐	No ☐
Is an activity that won't be easily blocked or prevented by practical problems?	Yes ☐	No ☐
Will help me to learn useful things, even if it doesn't work out perfectly?	Yes ☐	No ☐

You should be able to answer yes to each of the questions above. If your current plan has failed on one of the questions, try to think why this is so. What changes can you make to alter or improve it? Try to change things so that any poorly planned aspects are improved.

Part of this planning phase should include planning what you will do if your initial plan doesn't work out fully. What if it doesn't work out? Write here your plan of what you can do next:

....

....

....

In your activity diary, write down exactly **when you will do it**. Plan to do it this week so it is clear **when** you will put it into practice.

(e.g.) EXAMPLE

Anne's plan for tackling her reduced activity

Here are Anne's reflections on the six questions for effective change:

- **Will it be useful for understanding or changing how I am?** 'Even though I worry how the conversation will go, I think it will be useful for me to do this anyway. I think that is an important thing for me to change. It will get me back into contact again with someone I like.'

- **Is it a specific task so that I will know when I have done it?** 'I'm clear what I am going to do: I'll phone her up this evening. That way I'll definitely know whether I have done it.'

- **Is it realistic, practical and achievable?** 'Is it realistic? Yes, I can do that. I'd be lying if I didn't admit to myself that the idea of doing this scares me a bit. I don't know what she'll say to me. But it's really only a little bit scary. I am sure I can do this.'

- **Does it make clear what you are going to do and when you are going to do it?** 'I will phone her this evening, after 7 p.m. – she will be home from work then.'

- **Is it an activity that won't be easily blocked or prevented by practical problems?** 'Now then, what might block it? Maybe she won't be in when I phone. If so, I'll phone again later tonight or try again tomorrow. I am so worried that there may be some gaps in the conversation and that will be very embarrassing. I'll get around that by writing down three or four things we could cover in the conversation. I could ask her about the holiday – where she went, the hotel, the beaches and the food. I also really want to know about whether she had a good time and whether she met anyone there. I need to plan out how to ask that! The only other thing that I can predict could prevent me doing this is if I lose my nerve and try to put off calling her tonight, but I think it will be alright.'

- **Will it help me to learn useful things even if it doesn't work out perfectly?** 'Yes. I've come up with all sorts of ideas. If I do chicken out, then I'll know I need to do something slower first. Perhaps like writing or emailing first. I do think I can phone her though.'

Anne's goals are **clear** and **specific**, and her target is **realistic**. She knows **what** she is going to do and **when** she is going to do it. She has predicted potential difficulties that might get in the way. This seems like a well thought-through plan.

EXAMPLE

Harvinder's plan for tackling his avoidance

Harvinder uses the questions for effective change to help review his plan:

● **Will it be useful for understanding or changing how I am?** 'I can go to small local shops at the moment. I try to go at quieter times, like the early afternoon, and then rush round. If I could change that rushing around and still go to the shop, then that would be an important first step.'

● **Is it a specific task so that I will know when I have done it?** 'I need to be clear about what I am going to do. I will go shopping as I normally do. But instead of just shooting round the shop and grabbing the things I need, I will try to walk round it at a slower pace. I'll know I've done this if I look at my watch just before I go into the shop and again just after I leave. I want to stay in there at least ten minutes to begin with.'

● **Is it realistic, practical and achievable?** 'Is it realistic? Yes, I can do that. It's really only a little bit scary. I'm sure I can do this.'

● **Does it make clear what you are going to do and when you are going to do it?** 'I have a clear idea of what I need to do. I will spend at least ten minutes in the shop. I need to think about how I can spend the extra time there. I could look for some other provisions or read the ingredient labels. Even better: I could stop at the video stand and look at what videos they have in. That's something that could take a few minutes. I need to decide when I am going to do this trip to the shops. I think I should do it on Tuesday at 2 p.m.'

● **Is it an activity that won't be easily blocked or prevented by practical problems?** 'Now then, what might block it? If the shop was very busy, I might want to leave more quickly. I could plan to go at a quieter time of day, and even if there are a few people there I could choose to stay in. The only other thing that I can predict could prevent me doing this is if I lose my nerve and try to start rushing round when I get there. If I have that temptation, I just need to make sure I slow down my breathing and also my walking. I'll deliberately not leave the shop and just stay there for a few more minutes before leaving. I know from before that I'm going to notice my usual fear that "I will collapse". I need to be aware of that and try to challenge these fears.'

● **Will it help me to learn useful things even if it doesn't work out perfectly?** 'I'm pretty sure this will all be OK. But if it is too scary and I really can't cope, then I'll pick something less scary instead. At least I have other options on my list. I think I can do this though.'

Again, this is a well-planned approach.

Step 6: carry out the plan

Pay attention to your thoughts about what will happen before, during and after you have completed your plan.

 Write down any extreme and unhelpful thoughts you noticed. Record how much you believed them at the time, from 0% (not at all) to 100% (fully).

My thought(s):

....

....

....

I believed this   % **before** the task.

I believed this   % **during** the task.

I believed this   % **after** the task.

Record how anxious you felt at the time, from 0% (no anxiety) to 100% (maximum anxiety possible).

My level of anxiety:

% **before** the task.

% **during** the task.

% **after** the task.

Remember that as you carry out the plan, you are undermining your old fears by acting against them. There is the added bonus that you are also doing something that can give you a sense of achievement and pleasure.

(e.g.) EXAMPLE

Anne's plan

Anne phones Sarah that evening. Initially, Sarah is out and Anne has an immediate negative thought: 'I knew she'd be out. What's the point?' She believes this 80% and feels quite down. Anne thinks back to her plan and decides to do what she had planned if Sarah was out at first. Anne therefore phones back again later that evening and finds that Sarah is in. Sarah is delighted to hear from Anne, and they chat for over half an hour. They have so much to chat about that Sarah asks whether they can ring each other again the next day. Overall, Anne realises that she has gained some pleasure and a definite sense of achievement from the conversation and that her predictions about how it would go wrong were unfounded.

Harvinder's plan

Harvinder goes to the shop the next day. Before he enters the shop, he writes down his anxious thoughts on a piece of paper and records how much he believes them. He reminds himself that as he carries out the plan, this will help undermine the old fears. Before he goes into the shop, he notices the fear 'I will collapse.' He believes this 30% at the time. He records his anxiety as being 30% as well. He challenges it by reminding himself that he has never collapsed. When he goes into the shop, there are three other people in there – an older couple and a schoolchild. His belief that he will collapse shoots up to 80%. He rates himself as 70% anxious. He thinks about leaving and begins to feel hot and sweaty. He notices an increase in both his heart rate and his breathing. He begins to walk faster to try to get all his shopping done as quickly as possible. He then remembers that he had decided that if he felt like this, he would try to control

---

his breathing and slow down his walking. Harvinder makes a big effort and stops in the aisle by the videos. He picks one up and looks at the description on the back. He does this for a couple of minutes and begins to feel much better. His anxiety and belief that he will collapse both drop slowly to around 40%. He is able to complete the rest of his shopping at a normal pace. When he leaves the shop, he is surprised to find that he has been in there for almost 15 minutes.

Step 7: review the outcome

Write what happened here:

✎

....

....

....

Was the approach successful?	Yes ☐	No ☐
Did it help improve things?	Yes ☐	No ☐
Were there any disadvantages to using this approach?	Yes ☐	No ☐

(?) What have I learned from doing this? Write down any helpful lessons or information you have learned from what happened. If things didn't go quite as you hoped, try to learn from this. How could you make things different during your next attempt to tackle the problem?

✎

....

....

....

(e.g.) EXAMPLE

Anne's review

That went really well. I almost gave up when Sarah wasn't in. I'm really pleased that I stuck to the plan and phoned her back. We had a great chat. The two things I have learned are:

● Just how useful it is to have predicted that Sarah might not be in when I phoned. When that happened it was discouraging and I felt quite down. But I quickly challenged my initial negative reaction and phoned again.

● All my concerns about it being very embarrassing and anxiety-provoking weren't true. I did feel anxious when I got through to her, but I noticed that the anxiety quickly began to fall as I chatted to her.

Harvinder's review

That went generally well. I was almost thrown when there were three people already in the shop. That hardly ever happens. The three things I have learned are:

● Just how useful it is to have predicted what to do if I began to feel worse. When that happened, I felt really scared. I remembered that I had planned to slow down my breathing and my walking if that happened. It worked! I felt a lot better – especially after looking at the video.

● All my concerns about collapsing if I stayed in just weren't true. I did feel anxious when I went in – especially when I noticed the others there. However, the anxiety quickly began to fall as time passed. It didn't just keep going up and up like I thought it would.

● Although at the time when I felt most anxious, I believed the fears that 'I'm going to collapse', the fear and physical sensations did not continue rising. I didn't collapse and, when I think back, I never have collapsed while shopping. I certainly believe that I'll collapse far less than before.

By repeating the same activity **again and again** over the next week, Harvinder's fear becomes less and less intense. It also lasts for shorter and shorter lengths of time. By repeatedly facing his fears, he is able to challenge his fearful thoughts and reduce his anxiety as well as tackling his anxiety. This same pattern happens no matter what fear is being tackled. Facing up to a fear causes it to slowly lose its impact. This is illustrated in the diagrams below.

First time Harvinder faces his fears in the small local shop: Tuesday at 2pm.

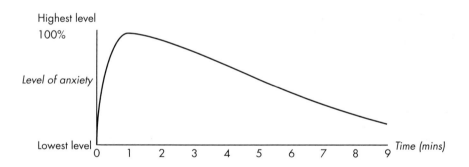

Second time when Harvinder faces his fears in the small local shop: Wednesday at 11.30am.

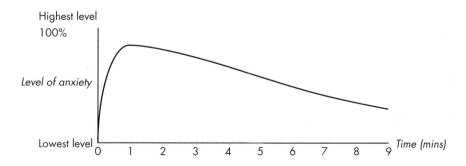

Third time when Harvinder faces his fears in the small local shop: Friday at 3pm.

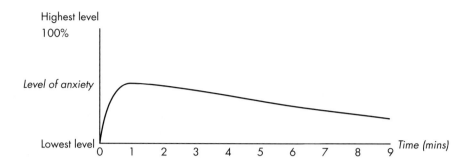

🔑 KEY POINT

By facing up to your fears, you can overcome them.

Putting into practice what you have learned

● Choose one or two areas of reduced activity or avoidance. Use the seven-step problem-solving approach during the next few days and weeks. Keep focused on changing just one problem area.

● After a week or so of trying this, read the final section of this workbook.

If you noticed problems with your plan

Choosing realistic targets for change is important. Were you too ambitious or unrealistic in choosing your target? Sometimes, a problem-solving approach may be blocked by something happening unexpectedly. Perhaps something didn't happen as you planned or someone reacted in an unexpected way? Try to learn from what happened.

(?) How could you change your approach to the problem and continue to apply the questions for effective change to help you create a realistic action plan?

✎

....

....

....

Section 4 Planning the next steps

Now that you have considered how your first planned activity went, the next step is to plan another activity to build on this. You need to think again about your **short-term**, **medium-term** and **longer-term** targets. Did your plan help you completely tackle the area of reduced activity or avoidance you were working on? You may need to plan out other solutions to tackle different aspects of your problem. The key is to build one step upon another.

For example, Harvinder has managed to go into a small local shop repeatedly. This has really helped him move things forward and has boosted his confidence. He still needs to keep working on tackling his problems, though, so that he can work up to successfully shopping in large shops such as supermarkets.

Steps should always be realistic, practical and achievable. Without this sort of step-by-step approach, you may find that although you take some steps forward, they are in different directions and you lose your focus and motivation as a result. Use what you have just learned to build on what you did.

Many people find this approach takes quite a lot of practice. It may also be tempting to be too ambitious. Remember, large changes can be achieved by moving one step at a time. By making slow sure steps, you will also boost your confidence and increase your sense of having the ability to deal with the problems you face.

You have the choice to:

- Repeat what you did.
- Take what you did and move it on one stage further.
- Or select a new area of activity from your checklists on pages 14–16.

Each of these choices has advantages and disadvantages. Think about what the advantages and disadvantages may be for you.

The key is to do everything at the right pace, so that change happens. It should not be so quickly that it seems too difficult to achieve. Slow sure steps forward are the best way to make progress.

Remember: repeat each step several times before moving on. The more times you can practise, the better. Doing this will boost your confidence in your ability to change. If you have any problems use the questions for effective change to plan the step again, or set a more realistic target.

Do:

- Continue to plan to alter **only one** area of activity or avoidance at a time.
- Break down the problem into smaller parts, each of which builds towards your eventual goal. There can be as many or as few steps as you want in your plan.
- Produce a plan to alter slowly what you do in an effective way.
- Be realistic in your goals.
- Use the questions for effective change to help plan each step.
- Write down your plan in detail so that you will be able to put it into practice this week.

If you find any step too difficult, **go back a stage and regain your confidence**. Then, decide on a different next step that is not quite so difficult. Repeat this step successfully several times before trying again with the step you found too difficult.

Don't:

- Choose something that is too ambitious a target to do next.

- Try to start to alter too many areas of your life all at once.
- Be very negative and think 'Nothing can be done.' Instead, try to experiment to find out whether this negative thinking is true or helpful.
- Try to move too quickly from one step to the next. Make sure you succeed repeatedly at each step first.

Most difficulties can be overcome using this approach. Remember that the main reason for a plan being ineffective is if you are too ambitious or allow yourself to believe that change is impossible.

Once you have chosen the next step you wish to change, write it down here:

✎

....

....

....

Use what you learned earlier to write your action plan. Plan **what** you will do and **when** you will do it. Learn from what happens so that you can keep putting into practice what you have learned. By doing this, you will slowly be able to rebuild your confidence and increase your feelings of pleasure and achievement.

Create a weekly action plan

Each week you can build these targets, one upon another. This will move you forwards one step at a time.

---

e.g. EXAMPLE

Anne's weekly plan

Anne's weekly targets	Timescale
Phone Sarah	Week 1
Contact other old friends and acquaintances by phone	Week 2
Arrange to meet up with Sarah at my flat	Week 3
Go for a curry with Sarah	Week 4
Arrange to meet a few people for a meal out at a restaurant	Weeks 5 and 6
Ultimate target: be able to have three or four friends round to my flat for a meal	Week 7

The key is to do everything at the right pace, so that change happens, but not so quickly that it seems too fast or too scary.

EXAMPLE

Harvinder's weekly plan

Harvinder plans out the different steps that he needs to complete over the next few weeks. His plan should also include reducing and stopping doing some of the more subtle types of avoidance he has noticed. In Harvinder's case, this is rushing around the shop and gripping hard on the trolley.

Harvinder's weekly targets	Initial fear level (0–100%)	Timescale
Going into the local shop for a paper. Walking round slowly, and staying there for at least 10 minutes	Hardly scary at all: 5–10% scary	Week 1, and then repeat at least twice
Going into the local shop. Deliberately choosing a busier time of day, and again walking round slowly, staying in the shop for at least 20 minutes each time	A little scary: 15% scary	Week 2, and then repeat at least twice
Queuing in the post office and deliberately choosing the longest queue	Quite scary: 35% scary	Week 3, and then repeat at least twice
Going into the supermarket foyer area to buy a newspaper and staying there for at least 20 minutes	Pretty scary: 50% scary	Weeks 4 and 5, and then repeat at least twice
Going into the supermarket at a quieter time and shopping for at least 20 minutes. Relaxing my grip on the trolley	Moderately scary: 75% scary	Week 6, and then repeat at least twice
Going shopping in the supermarket by myself at a busier time for at least 20 minutes. Having a relaxed grip on the trolley all the time	Very scary: 85% scary	Week 7, and then repeat at least twice
Ultimate target: going shopping in the supermarket by myself at a busier time and deliberately choosing the longest checkout queue. Spend at least 30 minutes in the shop	Very, very scary: 100% scary at first	Week 8, and then repeat at least twice

You can see that Harvinder's plan is in fact made up of a series of separate targets. **Each next target on the way can be planned out in detail using the seven-step approach.** Each new target builds upon the previous one to help Harvinder to move forwards. At each stage, he is able to test out and challenge his original fear further.

You can see that the steps taken are rated in terms of how scary and difficult they seem when Harvinder first creates the plan. The plan helps Harvinder to face up to his fear in a planned and paced way. This means that he never feels so anxious that he wants to give up. By repeating each new stage several times a week, Harvinder can build up his confidence before moving on to the next step. If he found that a particular stage is too difficult, he could always take a step back and re-plan the task. By succeeding in these planned steady steps, real progress can be achieved.

(task) Write out the next few weeks of your own step-by-step approach:

My step-by-step targets	Initial fear level (0–100%)	Timescale (weeks)

The key is to do everything at the right pace, so that change happens. Slow sure steps forward are the best way to make progress.

 IMPORTANT POINT

Repeat each step several times before moving on to the next step. The more times you can practise each step, the better. Doing this will boost your confidence in your ability to change. If you have any problems, use the questions for effective change to plan the step again, or set a more realistic target.

Practical hints and tips for boosting activity

● Copy the blank activity diary at the end of this workbook. Plan your activities to include a range of things that give you a sense of pleasure, achievement and confidence each week.

- Use the diary to plan to do something **for yourself** each day, e.g. reading, having a bath, listening to music, having a little treat or simply having time for yourself, even if only for a little time each day.

- Consider taking up something that you value, especially something that gives you a sense of purpose, e.g. voluntary work, helping tidy the local park, or helping a political, community or religious organisation. Can you help with the local school or plan to do a further education course that interests you? Could you join a club such as photography or bird-watching if you've enjoyed that in the past?

- Get in contact with people you like by letter, email or phone. Talk and listen more. Do things together. Don't focus overly on just one relationship. The workbook *Building relationships* can help you with this. If you find that you have been isolated for many years and it's difficult to think of who you might contact, switch to a problem-solving approach. Work through the workbook *Practical problem-solving* with this in mind.

- Write down some **goals** in a notebook at the start of the week and take satisfaction as you tick them off at the end of the week. At the end of the week, write down other things that you've achieved. Make sure that the goals are realistic and really can be resolved within that week.

- Finally, **exercise** can have an important and positive impact on many aspects of your life. A general increase in exercise is known to be associated with boosted mood, a healthier body and improved sleep. The benefits of exercise are now being recognised and many areas provide referral to physiotherapists and gyms to help boost mood and increase fitness levels. If you have symptoms that restrict you physically, then you can always discuss appropriate goals of fitness with your doctor or physiotherapist. In general, maintaining activities at the level you can cope with is a sensible option. You can find out more about how to do this in the workbook *Using exercise to boost how you feel*.

Section 5   **Workbook summary**

In this workbook, you have:
- Discovered how symptoms affect our lives.
- Identified any reduced activity and avoidance in your own life and considered the impact on you.
- Learned how to record your current activity levels.
- Seen examples of ways of overcoming reduced activity and avoidance.
- Practised this approach to make slow, steady changes to your life.
- Planned some next steps to build on this improvement.

Putting into practice what you have learned

Carry out a series of **action plans** over the next few weeks to tackle your avoidance and reduced activity. If you have difficulties, just do what you can.

Acknowledgements

I wish to thank all those who have commented upon this workbook, especially Dr Nicky Dummett and Catriona Kent.

Answer to Anne's example on pages 3–4.

Symptoms (Box 1)	Problems of arthritis years make it difficult for her to get out. Six months of worsening lower back pain. Feeling increasingly low and upset
Reduced total activity (Box 2)	She is generally doing far less
Reduced activity of valued things (Box 3)	She is no longer walking across to the park bench and seeing and chatting to people there. She has stopped listening to music and talk shows on the radio, and stopped reading. She has reduced contact with her brother and his children and she is increasingly isolated, sitting alone in her chair

Overall, this causes her to **feel worse** (Box 4).

My notes

....
....
....
....
....
....
....
....
....
....
....
....
....
....
....
....
....
....
....
....
....
....
....
....
....

My notes

....

Activity diary/planner

Date and time	Activity (include everything you do)	Duration (how long did you do it for?)	Pleasure felt (0 = no pleasure; 10 = maximum pleasure)	Sense of achievement gained (0 = no sense of achievement; 10 = maximum sense of achievement)
6–7 a.m.				
7–8 a.m.				
8–9 a.m.				
9–10 a.m.				
10–11 a.m.				
11–12 p.m.				
12–1 p.m.				
1–2 p.m.				
2–3 p.m.				
3–4 p.m.				

Activity diary/planner

Day and date	Activity (include everything you do)	Duration (how long did you do it for?)	Pleasure felt (0 = no pleasure; 10 = maximum pleasure)	Sense of achievement gained (0 = no sense of achievement; 10 = maximum sense of achievement)
4–5 p.m.				
5–6 p.m.				
6–7 p.m.				
7–8 p.m.				
8–9 p.m.				
9–10 p.m.				
10–11 p.m.				
11 p.m.–12 p.m.				
12 p.m.–1 a.m.				

Using exercise to boost how you feel

Dr Chris Williams

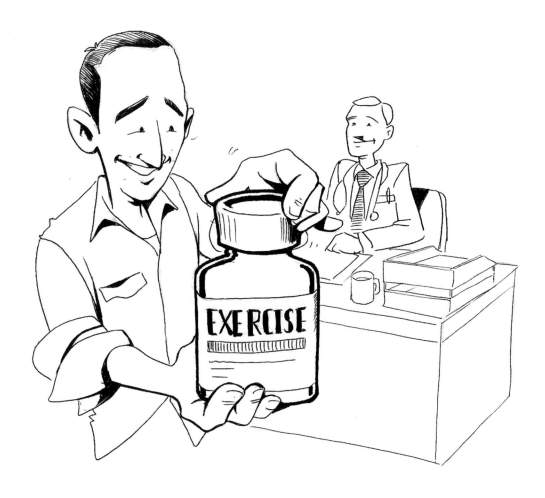

A Five Areas Approach
Helping you to help yourself
www.livinglifetothefull.com

Section 1   **Introduction**

In this workbook you will:
- Find out about the impact of activity and exercise on your mental and physical health.
- Learn how to use exercise to help you feel better.
- Do an experiment to discover the impact exercise can have on how you feel.
- Make a clear plan that works for you.
- Learn how to overcome stumbling blocks that can hold you back from making positive changes.

The impact of activity and exercise on our mental and physical health

Our emotions, thinking, behaviour, relationships, life situation and body all affect each other. Think about a time when you have had a bad cold. We have a runny nose and a sore throat, but also we can feel subdued, fed-up and emotionally down. The illness can affect us emotionally as well as physically. Likewise, physical activity can affect us emotionally – but this time in more helpful ways.

In contrast, think back to times in your life when you have exercised, such as riding a bike, playing football or going swimming. Some people find that as well as having the physical workout, they often notice a mental 'high' after exercise. In the past, many of the main treatments used for problems with low or anxious mood were based on exercise. Exercise may now be 'prescribed' by many doctors as part of a treatment package for depression.

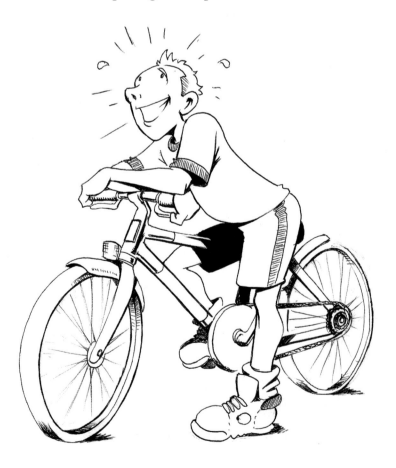

Using exercise to help you feel better

Planned exercise has been shown to boost mood, reduce tension and anxiety, and improve self-esteem – as well as helping us become physically fitter.

Other benefits include:

- It can be fun, if you choose something that you have previously liked doing.
- It gives **you** control. You are in charge and can plan things at your own pace.
- It can help you structure and plan your day – you set up new habits rather than just staying in and being inactive.
- It can boost your social life. Doing things with others such as an aerobics class or a walking group can help you meet other people with a shared interest.
- There are wider long-term benefits, such as reducing your risk of high blood pressure, stroke and heart attacks. It can have a helpful role in preventing the bone problem osteoporosis. Finally, it reduces the risk of diabetes.

Exercise really is a win–win situation.

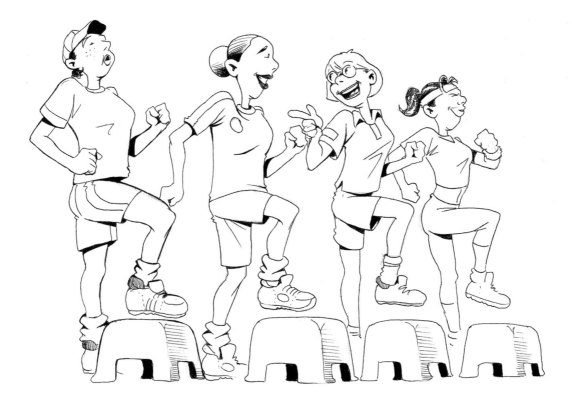

However, there are a number of challenges and difficulties in becoming more active:

- There can be side effects, e.g. aching muscles.
- You may have to pay for some activities, e.g. for using a gym or swimming pool.

 EXPERIMENT

You will need less than 15 minutes to do this experiment. The aim is to test out whether even a small amount of exercise affects how you feel emotionally.

Before you start, think of a physical activity that you can do. This should be something that:

- Can be done in just five to ten minutes to start with.

- Is realistic, bearing in mind how physically fit you are at the moment.

● You know is within your capabilities and doesn't push you. Choose something that doesn't involve vigorous exercise. This isn't asking you to do a workout – you don't need to get changed, work up a sweat or even do warm-up exercises.

For example, walk up and down the stairs three or four times. Take a rest if you get out of breath (like the author, who makes no claims to fitness!). Other things you might try are to stretch your body, jog slowly on the spot or walk around the block at a reasonable pace. Don't pick too ambitious a target – we're not looking for a marathon here. If you are physically unwell, you can always check this with your doctor first if you have any concerns.

You've chosen what to do. Now, **before you start**, put a cross on the two lines below to show how you feel **right now**:

Sadness/happiness

Very sad	OK	Very happy

Tension/anxiety

Very tense/anxious	OK	Very relaxed

Next, carry out your five to ten minutes of minor exercise, stopping for a rest if you feel this is too long for you.

Immediately afterwards, re-rate your mood:

Sadness/happiness

Very sad	OK	Very happy

Tension/anxiety

Very tense/anxious	OK	Very relaxed

Next, **stop, think and reflect**. Have a look back at your scores before and after. Did you notice any changes? How did you feel during the task? Remember: any benefits can be boosted even more by planning to do activities that are fun.

Write down any changes you noticed in your thoughts/mental energy/how positive you feel/your ability to think clearly:

✎

....

....

....

Write down any changes you noticed in how you felt emotionally, e.g. tension, anger, stress, sadness, happiness, enthusiasm:

✎

....

....

....

Write down any changes you noticed in how you felt physically, e.g. relaxed/tense, jittery, tired, achy, ready for more:

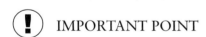

....

....

....

Write down any other changes you noticed:

....

....

....

(?) **Overall**, do you think you might benefit from planning in some exercise into your life as part of your own mental-fitness package?　　Yes ☐　　No ☐

　Many people find that exercise does bring benefits. The improvements through exercise can boost how we feel and activate us into making more use of these workbooks. We know that making positive changes in one area can bring benefits to the other areas.

Yes, but . . .

There are lots of things in life that we know are good for us, but still we don't do them. That is just as true in the author's life as it may be in your own. Often, the biggest problems are simple ones:

● We just aren't in the habit of doing exercise.
● We want to get into the habit, but it proves hard. For example, it's easy for us to talk ourselves out of something. This is especially true with issues such as exercise, because for many of us exercise is seen as **too hard, boring, expensive** or **too time-consuming** – or all of these.

(!) IMPORTANT POINT

We could spend quite a lot of time here looking at ways of challenging thoughts that exercise is too hard, boring or time-consuming. If you have these thoughts, use the workbook *Identifying and changing extreme and unhelpful thinking* to look at ways of overcoming these sorts of blocking thoughts. In the meantime, please do choose to exercise – it can make a real difference to how you feel. Exercise can be as effective as medication, but with fewer side effects. It may be hard, but you can slowly set up new habits.

Exercise and injury

One of the benefits of seeing a professional such as a physiotherapist, personal trainer or gym worker is that they can help you to plan a fitness programme appropriate for you. They can also advise you on how to **warm up in order to avoid muscle pulls, aches and strains**. Using good techniques and the right equipment, clothing and footwear is important.

Keeping a balance

Because exercise can sometimes give people a real buzz, there can be a danger that the amount of exercise builds up and up in an addictive way. Try to seek the right balance here. If you know you are an all-or-nothing type of person, try to rein in your tendency to overdo it by sticking to a balanced plan.

Medication and exercise

Remember that other approaches for low mood and tension such as medication can be used alongside exercise. If you are riding a bike on the road or doing any exercises where reaction times and judgement are needed, be aware that medication can sometimes make you feel drowsy. In general, if the label or information leaflet with your medication urges you to be cautious when operating machinery or driving a car, then this will apply to cycling and other sports as well. Discuss your exercise plan with your doctor if you are in any doubt.

Section 2   **Making a clear plan that works for you**

People are often amazed at how empowering, energising and good it can feel when they get into a new habit of using exercise as part of their regular day.

You know you – your available time and what you like and dislike. All of this needs to be taken into account in your plan.

- Choose something that gets you going physically. Build up the amount of exercise slowly in a gradual and planned way.
- Don't throw yourself into things too quickly – or start too slowly. **Pacing is the key.**
- Many people find that doing exercise at the start of the day helps them get going. However, you need to be realistic. For example, if you have young children, then later in the day may be a better choice. Try to avoid exercising just before going to bed, as this can unhelpfully affect your sleep.
- Start exercising with help. **Structured and supervised exercise** treatment is often available 'on prescription' from your doctor. Exercise treatment can also be offered by, for example, physiotherapists and occupational therapists. If a local scheme isn't available, then perhaps you could devise your own plan with gym staff or a health practitioner.
- The course at www.livinglifetothefull.com offers you the chance to have short **monthly email reminders** to help keep you on track. This is free and you can cancel at any time. Please note, however, that we cannot offer any advice on an individual basis.

Overcoming blocks to change

If you really can't bring yourself to be enthusiastic about doing exercise, then perhaps you could choose to view it as a 'treatment'. We often talk about experiments in these workbooks. If you really aren't sure that exercise will work, you can test it out.

Planning when and how to exercise

Exercising on a regular basis – even if it is just a short time to begin with – is important. It is often helpful to actively plan this into your day and diary rather than just trying to fit it in at some time. Decide how long it should take to notice changes to your health and wellbeing. For example, after doing the same exercise for two weeks, you should find you can do it for slightly longer or go slightly further in the same amount of time. This can lead to a real sense of achievement and show that you are getting fitter.

You may find the following task helpful in making this regular commitment. Use it to help you plan how to exercise over the next week.

My plan to use exercise to help me feel better

What am I going to do? Remember to choose something that is possible, realistic and achievable. Preferably choose something that is fun. Consider planning in some exercise that has a social aspect at least once a week, e.g. an aerobics class or going for a run or walk with some friends. Remember that exercise doesn't need to cost lots of money. Exercise videos and DVDs are available for a small weekly charge from your local library. Or you could walk to your local shop each time instead of taking the bus or driving.

....
....
....

When am I going to plan to do some exercise? Is every day practical? If so, at what time of day? If not every day, then how about just once or twice a week? You can always build upon this at a later stage.

....
....
....

How much will I do? Be realistic, based on your current fitness levels, health and motivation. If in doubt about your health, discuss this with your doctor first.

....
....
....

Is this **realistic**, practical and achievable? You know your own life and its various demands and commitments.

....
....
....

What **problems** or **difficulties** could block or prevent me from doing this, e.g. children, money, work or health problems, and how can I overcome them?

✎

....

....

....

Write your plan into the activity planner at the end of this workbook. As you exercise, rate your feelings of pleasure and achievement using the scale on the sheet. You may wish to put your plan in a place where you will see it every day as a reminder.

Keeping on track

Once you have created your exercise plan, it is important to keep on track. This involves setting yourself goals and reviewing your progress. This allows you to make changes if things aren't going well.

(task)

My plan for the next few weeks

Consider short-, medium- and long-term changes:

What are you going to do?

✎

....

....

....

How will you try to make sure that you carry out your plan?

✎

....

....

....

When are you going to do it?

✎

....

....

....

What can **stop this happening**? What problems and difficulties might there be, and how can you overcome them? What might sabotage your plan?

✎

....

....

....

Apply the questions for effective change to your plan. Is your planned task one that:

Will be useful for understanding or changing how you are?	Yes ☐	No ☐
Is a specific task, so that you will know when you have done it?	Yes ☐	No ☐
Is realistic, practical and achievable?	Yes ☐	No ☐
Makes clear what you are going to do and when you are going to do it?	Yes ☐	No ☐
Is an activity that won't be easily blocked or prevented by practical problems?	Yes ☐	No ☐
Will help you learn useful things, even if it doesn't work out perfectly?	Yes ☐	No ☐

Date of my next review:

✎

....

....

....

Review your plan monthly. Set aside a time to do this – put it into your schedule or diary.

Section 3 **Workbook summary**

In this workbook you have learned:
- About the impact of activity and exercise on our mental and physical health.
- How to use exercise to help you feel better.
- Whether exercise can have an impact on how you feel.
- How to make a clear plan that works for you.
- How to overcome stumbling blocks that can hold us back from making positive changes.

Exercise is only one way to bring about change. Making changes to other aspects of your life can also make a big difference.

Putting into practice what you have learned

- Read through this workbook again and think about how you can use exercise to boost how you feel in all aspects of your life.
- Keep planning and reviewing your progress. At the same time, keep a balance so that you do the right level of exercise that is appropriate for your own life.

Acknowledgements

I wish to thank all those who have commented upon this workbook, especially Marie Chellingsworth, Catriona Kent, Eileen Riddoch and Dr Philip Wilson.

Exercise planner: my day

Date and time	Activity (include everything you do)	Duration (how long will you do it for?)	Pleasure felt (0 = no pleasure; 10 = maximum pleasure)	Sense of achievement gained (0 = no sense of achievement; 10 = maximum sense of achievement)
Morning				
Afternoon				
Evening				

Helpful and unhelpful things we can do

Dr Chris Williams

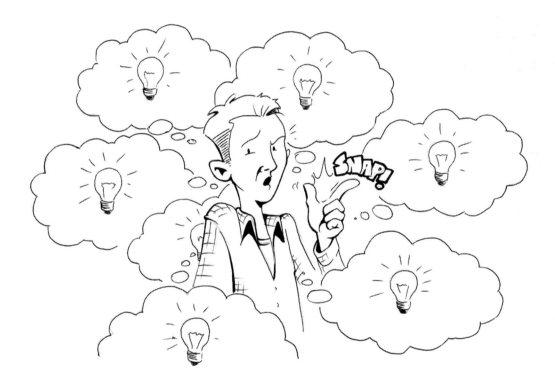

A Five Areas Approach
Helping you to help yourself
www.livinglifetothefull.com

Section 1   **Introduction**

In this workbook you will:
- Learn about helpful and unhelpful ways of responding to symptoms.
- Discover key information about the vicious circle of unhelpful behaviours.
- Learn some brief hints and tips of ways to reduce unhelpful behaviours.
- Practise a structured approach to plan a reduction in an unhelpful behaviour.

Helpful and unhelpful behaviours

When somebody experiences symptoms, it is normal that they try to do things to feel better. This altered behaviour may be **helpful** or **unhelpful**. The purpose is to help the person feel better.

Helpful activities may include things you can do yourself and things you can do with others, such as:
- Talking and receiving support from friends or relatives.
- Reading or using self-help materials so that you can find out more about the causes and treatment of the problems.
- Maintaining activities that provide pleasure or support, such as meeting friends, joining a group or attending a class.
- Challenging anxious thoughts by stopping, thinking and reflecting rather than accepting them as true.
- Going to see your doctor or healthcare practitioner or attending a self-help support group.

(task) Write here any **helpful** things you have done:

✎

....

....

....

....

....

You should aim to try to maximise the number of helpful activities you do as part of your recovery plan. By planning these helpful activities, this can boost how you feel.

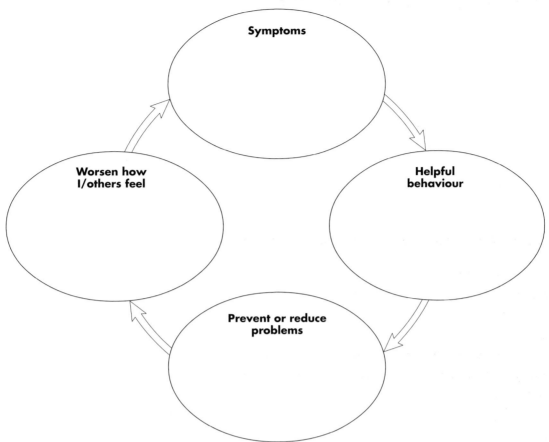

The circle of helpful behaviour

Checklist: identifying the circle of helpful behaviour

Am I:	Tick here if you have noticed this, even if only sometimes

Being good to myself, e.g. eating regularly and healthily, taking time to enjoy my food?

Doing things for fun and pleasure, e.g. hobbies, listening to music, having a nice bath?

Seeking support from others and sharing concerns appropriately with trusted friends and family members?

Seeking out other helpful sources of support, e.g. attending a voluntary-sector self-help group?

Socialising at a level I can cope with, whether by telephone or email or going out?

Stopping, thinking and reflecting on things rather than jumping to conclusions, and letting upsetting thoughts 'just be' rather than constantly mulling them over?

Finding out more, such as by reading self-help materials and other informative resources and putting into practice what I have learned?

Am I: **Tick here if you have noticed this, even if only sometimes**

Pacing myself and letting others know I am doing this, e.g. telling relatives I am planning to do less?

Keeping as active as I can, e.g. doing exercise, going for walks, swimming, pottering around the garden or going to a gym?

Using my sense of humour to cope?

Planning time for me as well as for others?

Taking any prescribed medication regularly and as prescribed?

Using effective coping responses such as relaxation techniques to deal with feelings of tension (see www.livinglifetothefull.com)?

Seeing a healthcare practitioner for advice, viewing recovery as an active and joint collaboration, and being honest with them about progress or when I feel stuck?

In situations with problems of pain, keeping active as much as possible and walking with as relaxed and normal a posture as possible?

(?) Am I doing any other helpful behaviour? Write in what you are doing here if this applies to you.

....

....

....

Having completed these questions, reflect on your answers using the three questions below:

Am I doing any activities or behaviours that improve how I feel?	Yes ☐	No ☐	Sometimes ☐
Are these activities/behaviours definitely helpful in the short and longer term for me or for others?	Yes ☐	No ☐	Sometimes ☐
Overall, has this improved how I/others feel?	Yes ☐	No ☐	Sometimes ☐

If you have answered yes or sometimes to all three questions, then you are responding in some helpful ways. You should try to build these helpful responses into your life.

(!) IMPORTANT POINT

Sometimes we can think that a behaviour is helpful when in fact it is part of the problem. Typical examples are patterns of drinking excessive alcohol, avoidance and reassurance-seeking. Each of these may well cause you to feel better in the short term (which is why they can be mistaken as helpful). However, in the medium and long term, they backfire and worsen how you or others feel in some way (physically, mentally or in your relationships). In contrast, a hallmark of a truly helpful activity is that it is good for you and often for others as well.

Unhelpful behaviours

Sometimes we try to block how we feel with a number of **unhelpful behaviours,** such as drinking too much alcohol in order to block how we feel, becoming very dependent on others or pushing people away. These actions often make us feel better in the short term. However, they can also backfire and create further problems. This can include immediate or longer-term negative impacts. These actions therefore act to keep the difficulties going and become part of the problem. A **vicious circle of unhelpful behaviour** may result.

The vicious circle of unhelpful behaviour

Symptoms/
problems

Unhelpful
behaviour
e.g. drinking too much
alcohol, becoming very
dependent

Worsen how
I/others feel

Create or worsen
problems

 Look at the following list and tick any activity you have found yourself doing in the past few weeks. A wide range of different unhelpful behaviours has been summarised here to help you to think about changes that could be happening in your own life.

As a result of how I feel, am I:	Tick here if you have noticed this, even if only sometimes
Misusing alcohol, illegal drugs or prescribed medication to block how I feel in general or improve how I sleep?	
Eating too much to block how I feel ('comfort eating') or overeating so much that this becomes bingeing?	
Making impulsive decisions about important things, e.g. resigning a job without really thinking through the consequences?	
Being overly aware and checking excessively for symptoms of ill health?	
Setting myself up to fail?	

As a result of how I feel, am I: **Tick here if you have noticed this, even if only sometimes**

Trying to spend my way out of how I feel by going shopping ('retail therapy')?

Becoming very demanding or excessively seeking reassurance from others?

Using television soaps or the Internet to block how I feel and substitute for other relationships around me?

Looking to others to make decisions or sort out problems for me?

Setting myself up to be rejected by others?

Throwing myself into doing things, so I am so busy that there are no opportunities to stop, think and reflect?

Pushing others away and being verbally or physically threatening or rude to them?

Deliberately harming myself in an attempt to block how I feel?

Doing risk-taking actions, e.g. crossing the road without looking or gambling using money I don't really have?

Compulsively checking, cleaning or doing things a set number of times or in exactly the 'correct' order so as to make things 'right'?

Carrying out mental rituals such as counting or deliberately thinking 'good thoughts' to make things feel 'right'?

Sleeping with various people as a means of blocking how I feel or to prove my attractiveness/worth?

If you are noticing physical pain: excessively changing the way I sit or walk in order to reduce symptoms of physical discomfort? The altered posture then creates or worsens the physical problem.

Having completed these questions, reflect on your answers using the three questions below:

Am I doing certain activities or behaviours that are designed to improve how I feel?	Yes ☐	No ☐	Sometimes ☐
Are some of these activities unhelpful in the short or longer term, either for me or for others?	Yes ☐	No ☐	Sometimes ☐
Overall, has this worsened how I feel?	Yes ☐	No ☐	Sometimes ☐

If you have answered yes or sometimes to all three questions, then you are experiencing a pattern of unhelpful behaviour.

Let's now look at some examples of how these behaviours backfire and worsen things.

EXAMPLE

Paul's drinking

Paul has been off work for a number of months and has developed money worries. He is also concerned whether he will ever get back to work. He has started to drink more alcohol to try and cope. This is now affecting both him and his wife Sally. Look at how this is affecting him.

Paul's drinking (vicious circle of unhelpful behaviour)

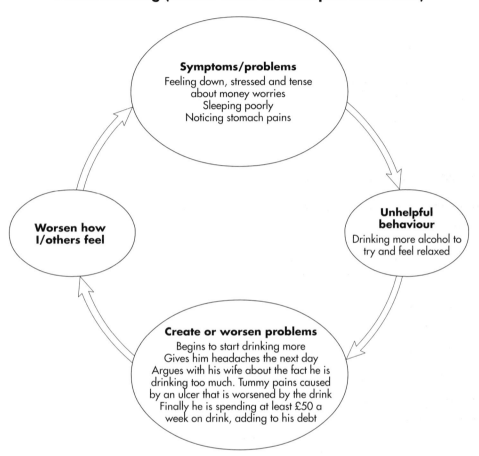

Paul does not think he has a drink problem. Instead, he sees alcohol as something that is helpful. This is because he hasn't worked out the unhelpful impact of alcohol on him. He needs to start looking at the downsides of the drinking as well as the immediate benefits. This means looking at the short- and longer-term consequences of his daily drinking for both him and other people.

What impact does the drinking have on Paul and Sally?

Short-term:

● **Physically:** headaches, hungover the next day, bad stomach pains.

● **Psychologically:** helps me sleep at night to begin with, makes me feel more relaxed, but then I wake up and have to go to the loo.

● **Socially:** makes me more likely to swear at Sally when she says she is worried about my drinking.

Longer-term (just one year later):

● **Physically:** Paul's stomach ulcer bursts; he is admitted to hospital and needs an emergency operation.

● **Psychologically:** alcohol can work as a chemical depressant: it causes anxiety and lowers mood. Paul becomes increasingly anxious, angry and depressed.

● **Socially:** Paul tries to return to work but his boss realises he is drinking too much and not coping. Paul loses his job. Sally cannot cope with how Paul is. They have more and more arguments. Finally, she leaves.

 EXAMPLE

Patrick's vicious circle of unhelpful behaviour

After a mild heart attack, Patrick is convinced that his heart is not working properly. As a result, he constantly feels anxious and is preoccupied with his illness. He pays special attention to the speed of his pulse and to any twinges of pain in his chest, whatever the cause. He constantly asks his wife Joyce how he looks.

Patrick's heart (vicious circle of unhelpful behaviour)

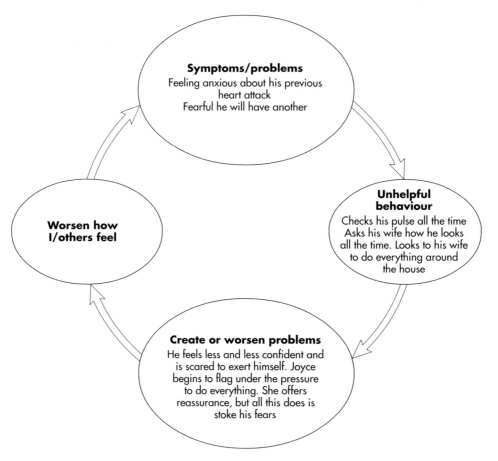

What impact does the reassurance-seeking have on Patrick and Joyce?

Short-term:

● **Physically and psychologically:** whenever Patrick feels anxious, his heart speeds up. Asking Joyce how he looks and hearing he is fine makes him feel less tense.

● **Socially:** to begin with, Joyce is concerned and wants to reassure Patrick that he looks well.

Longer-term:

● **Physically:** Patrick is unable to do his cardiac rehabilitation programme because of his avoidance of activity.

● **Psychologically:** Patrick becomes dependent on Joyce and looks to her to do everything for him.

● **Socially:** Joyce begins to struggle. She cannot cope with caring for Patrick, looking after the house, shopping and trying to keep her part-time job going. Eventually she sees her doctor to ask for an antidepressant.

(!) IMPORTANT POINT

Helpful and **unhelpful** behaviours are done because in the short term they make us feel better. The key difference is that in the longer term, unhelpful behaviours backfire and worsen how we or others feel. They become part of the problem. The good news is that if this applies to you, you can make changes.

Think about any examples of unhelpful behaviours you do. What impact do they have on you and those around you in the short and longer term?

Choose just one example of an unhelpful behaviour and write down its impact. What impact does the unhelpful behaviour have on you and those around you in the short term?

Physically:

....

....

....

Psychologically:

....

....

....

Socially (on you and others):

✎

....

....

....

And in the longer term:

Physically:

✎

....

....

....

Psychologically:

✎

....

....

....

Socially (on you and others):

✎

....

....

....

How our relationships with those around us can sometimes backfire

Let's think about the relationship between Joyce and Patrick in the example above. When we are feeling unwell, it can be a great resource, encouragement and help having family and friends around us who can offer support and a listening ear. What is needed is a balanced supportive relationship.

However, sometimes people around us may offer 'helpful advice' all the time and want to do **everything** for us. There can be many reasons for this. Often the cause is concern, friendship and love for us. Sometimes it may be the result of anxiety or, occasionally, guilt.

Whatever the cause, when others offer too much help and want to do everything for us, their actions can backfire in several ways:

- Their special attention may feel suffocating and frustrating. We can end up feeling as if we are being treated like a child. Arguments and little irritations build up and are upsetting to us both.
- Although they mean well, their actions can actually undermine how we feel. When trying to cope with symptoms, it is important to continue to do as many things as you are able to do within the confines of how you feel. If others take responsibility for doing everything for you, the danger is that you will not be as active as you could be. This can also damage your confidence. You will find out later that this can play a role in worsening how you feel.

Section 2   **Overcoming unhelpful behaviours**

By working through the seven steps outlined below, you can learn an approach that will help you to plan clear ways of overcoming any unhelpful behaviour.

Step 1: identify and define the problem to be tackled as precisely as possible

 EXAMPLE

Paul's drinking

Paul is drinking far more alcohol than he used to. This varies between spirits, wine and beer. He realises that his drinking is doing him harm, and he is fed up with the stomach pains he has noticed. He is also upset by the fact that he and Sally are constantly arguing about his drinking. She has left him once before and has now come back, but things are still tense. He decides he wants to **do something about it**.

Paul's first task is to find out exactly how much of a problem his drinking is at the moment. He therefore keeps a **drinking diary** to record his drinking over a one-week period in order to define his current drinking. He uses the blank drinking diary at the end of the workbook *Alcohol, drugs and you* and adds up the units he has each day. This confirms that he is drinking about 60 units a week. This is a surprise to Paul: he had thought he was drinking much less than this.

Paul decides that his **medium-term** target is to **reduce his drinking to only 20 units a week in two months' time**. He needs to write a clear step-by-step plan that is likely to be successful.

To do this, he needs to decide on a **realistic first step to take**. He sees his doctor and together they agree that his first step should be to reduce his drinking to 42 units a week.

Paul's initial target: 'I want to reduce my drinking to 42 units a week to begin with.'

Is this a good first target? Paul answers the next question to think about this further:

 Is this a small, focused problem that I can tackle in one step?   Yes ☑   No ☐

Paul has therefore broken down the problem into a **smaller target** that he can tackle first.

Step 2: think up as many solutions as possible to achieve your initial goal

It can sometimes seem difficult to even start tackling the problem. One way around this is to try to step back and see whether any other solutions are possible. This approach is called **brainstorming**. The more solutions that are generated, the more likely it is that a good one will emerge. The purpose of brainstorming is to try to come up with as many ideas as possible. Among them you hope to be able to identity a realistic, practical and achievable solution towards overcoming your problem.

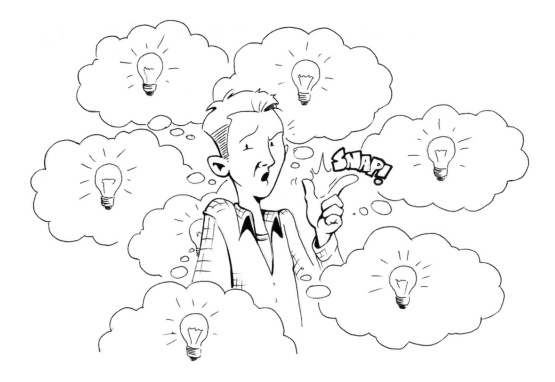

 EXAMPLE

Paul's brainstorming

● I could stop drinking completely on weekdays and have all 42 units at the weekend.

● I could plan to have, say, two units every night on the weekdays, and 32 units at the weekend.

● I could plan to drink the same amount each night, i.e. drink six units a night.

● I could join Alcoholics Anonymous and just stop drinking!

Step 3: look at the advantages and disadvantages of each possible solution

The next step is to think about the pros and cons of each option.

Suggestion	Advantages	Disadvantages
I could stop drinking completely on weekdays and have all 42 units at the weekend	My body could recover for five days. I could still have a night out with the lads	I know if I have a night out with the lads I'll blow it and drink loads. I'll really have some grief then from Sally. For the moment, I'm better off not going out. My doctor advised not to stop drinking suddenly or I might have some withdrawal problems. That means stopping drinking on weekdays isn't a good idea

Suggestion	Advantages	Disadvantages
I could plan to have, say, two units every night on the weekdays, and 32 units at the weekend	That still adds up to 42 units. I could have a bit of a drink every day. It would mean I wouldn't miss the drink or have withdrawal problems	I'm just a bit worried if I start drinking more at the weekend I'll just keep drinking. I know what I'm like
I could plan to drink the same amount each night, i.e. drink six units a night	I like this idea. It would keep everything nice and stable. There wouldn't be any big nights with lots of drinking. Sally would probably like that	It might feel quite boring. Just the same each night. It also means the weekend wouldn't be special. I suppose I could also have some alcohol-free beers as well if I went out
I could join Alcoholics Anonymous and just stop drinking!	Others might encourage me to give up. It would be good to know I'm not on my own	That doesn't fit my plan of aiming for 20 units a week in two months. I don't want to stop drinking completely

Step 4: choose one of the solutions

The chosen solution should be an option that will make a sensible first step in achieving your goal. It should be **realistic** and **likely to succeed**. The decision needs to be based on all the answers to step 3.

Paul decides on the third option (drinking the same amount each night) and to do this with help and advice from his healthcare practitioner. This solution should be an option that fulfils the following criteria:

Will it be **useful** for changing how you are?	Yes ☑	No ☐
Is it a **clear** task so you will know when you have done it?	Yes ☑	No ☐
Is it **realistic**, practical and achievable?	Yes ☑	No ☐

Other suggestions might also have worked, but this suggestion seems the most reasonable solution for Paul.

Step 5: plan the steps needed to carry it out

Paul's plan: 'I will cut my daily intake to six units every night. I won't have any days where I don't drink at all.' Paul also makes sure that as part of his plan he builds in some thought on what helpful things he could do even if his plan does not succeed fully.

Paul thinks about how he can apply the questions for effective change in deciding on his plan:

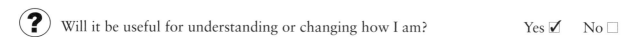 Will it be useful for understanding or changing how I am?   Yes ☑   No ☐

'Yes. If I use the right plan, I could learn that I can cut down my drinking.'

(?) Is it a specific task, so that I will know when I have done it?　　　Yes ☑　No ☐

'I'm clear what I am going to do – I want to have cut down to just 42 units a week. That will be my target and I'll spread the reduction in what I drink over the whole week. That's six units a night. I'll plan to drink wine or beer and stay off the spirits. I won't even keep spirits in the house, so I'm not tempted.'

(?) Is it realistic, practical and achievable?　　　Yes ☑　No ☐

'Yes. I could do this. I don't want to stop drinking completely, but that seems realistic. I know from what my doctor told me that if I try to stop all at once I'll probably not succeed, and also I might have some problems of alcohol withdrawal – I don't want that.'

(?) Does it make clear **what** you are going to do and **when** you are going to do it?　　　Yes ☑　No ☐

'I know what I'm going to do. I'll start tomorrow.'

(?) Is it an activity that won't be easily blocked or prevented by practical problems?　　　Yes ☑　No ☐

'What could prevent this? I'm due to go to Bob's party next Saturday. There's bound to be drinking there – I'd need to set myself a limit on that day. I may have fewer than six units because I'm driving. I also need to stop buying in six-packs for the time being – they are too tempting. The most I'll buy now is three cans a day (six units). That should help because I know that when I've had a few cans, I am often tempted to have a few more.'

(?) Will it help me to learn useful things even if it doesn't work out perfectly?　　　Yes ☑　No ☐

Paul can answer yes to each of these questions. If he couldn't, then he would need to think about what changes he could make to alter or improve his plan.

(!) IMPORTANT POINT

Part of this planning phase should include Paul having a planned response of how to react if his plan doesn't work out. Paul writes his response here:

'If it doesn't work out, I'll be definitely disappointed. If I have problems then at least I'll have learned what my "weak" times are for drinking. That way I can learn from this and take it into account with my future plans. My doctor says to expect occasional hiccups.'

Step 6: carry out the plan

Paul manages to put his plan into action for the first few days and he feels quite good about himself and how things are going. Things don't go according to plan, though, when he goes to Bob's party. He drinks two cans and then thinks 'What the heck? Let your hair down!' He ends up drinking ten pints of beer in a binge and has to take a taxi home. He has a blazing row with Sally and they end up sleeping in separate bedrooms. The next day Paul wakes up feeling worse and thinks about giving up his planned reduction in drinking completely. After a few hours, he begins to think about what he has learned before from his doctor about having to stick to a clear plan if he is going to succeed. He remembers his doctor telling him that it is likely there will be occasional hiccups, but that can still work out for the good. He can learn from what happens and plan to avoid making the same mistake again. Just because a setback occurs doesn't mean that everything is over. Paul therefore tries again and restarts his plan. With Sally's help he is able to succeed in reducing his drinking and reaches a limit of 42 units a week.

Step 7: review the outcome

Paul writes what happened here:

'Things have gone quite well. I managed to get down to 15 pints over the second week of trying. There was that major problem at Bob's party, but I've managed to overcome that. Just because a setback occurs does not mean that everything is over.'

Was the selected approach successful?	Yes ✓	No ☐
Did it help me to tackle the target problem?	Yes ✓	No ☐
Were there any disadvantages to using this approach?	Yes ☐	No ✓

(?) What have I learned from doing this?

'Try to stick to the plan. If things go wrong, don't give up but try to adjust so that you get back on target. Other people can really help – Sally's been fantastic.'

The example used shows how the technique might be applied to Paul's situation. However, it can also be applied to alter **any** unhelpful activity.

Planning the next steps

Paul's **medium-term** target is to **reduce his drinking to 20 units a week over the next two months.** He needs to have a clear step-by-step plan that is likely to be successful. He therefore needs to plan out the next steps to take after this first step.

EXAMPLE

Paul's strategy

Problem behaviour: drinking too much alcohol

	Units/week*	Time
Drinking 6 units a day every day	42 units	Week 1
Drinking 10 units at the weekend and 20 spread over the weekdays	30 units	Week 3
Drinking 10 units at the weekend and 14 units spread over the weekdays	24 units	Week 6
Drinking 10 units at the weekend, and 10 units spread over the weekdays	20 units	Week 8

*Note: one unit of alcohol is generally the same as a glass of wine, a single short such as whisky, or half a pint of beer. So one pint of beer contains about two units of alcohol. These estimates vary depending on the strength of the drink.

Target drinking level: 20 units a week.

Paul then uses the seven-step approach to plan each step so that he has a clear written plan of what he will do each week. He finds that he is able to reach his target over the next two months.

 KEY POINT

Paul's medium-term plan is in fact made up of a number of separate steps – in this case, four steps. Each step can be planned out in detail using the same seven-step approach. Each step builds on the previous steps to help Paul move forwards. Over a number of weeks, this can add up to a very significant total change in what Paul is able to achieve.

You now have the opportunity to try this approach yourself.

Section 3 Overcoming your own unhelpful behaviour

Apply what you have learned from Paul's example and use the questions below to help you to work through the seven-step approach to reducing your own unhelpful behaviour.

Look back at the checklist of unhelpful behaviours you completed on pages 5–6. From this, decide on an area of unhelpful behaviour you want to change.

Step 1: identify and define the problem as precisely as possible

It is not possible to deal with all your problems all at once. In fact, if you try to change everything at once, potentially you will be setting yourself up to fail. This is particularly important if you have ticked a number of boxes in the checklist. It is not possible to overcome all these areas at once. Select **only one problem area** that you wish to change at the present time.

Once you have chosen **one** target problem area, write it down here:

....
....
....

To begin with, record your unhelpful behaviour over several days. Make a written note of:

- When the behaviour or activity occurs.
- How much and how often you carry out this behaviour or activity, e.g. how many units of alcohol you drink, how many times you've sought reassurance, etc.
- How long it lasts for.

Use this information to help you to identify clearly the unhelpful behaviour that needs to be changed. Look back to Paul's example if you need help, or discuss it with a friend or your healthcare practitioner.

Ask yourself whether you need to break down this problem area into a number of smaller, more achievable targets. If so, write your first target here:

....
....
....

(?) Is this a small, focused problem that I can tackle in one step?   Yes ☐   No ☐

Step 2: think up as many solutions as possible to achieve your initial goal

Think about things you can do to overcome your chosen reduced activity. The purpose of brainstorming is to try to come up with as many ideas as possible. Among them you hope to be able to identity a realistic, practical and achievable solution. Completely wacky ideas should be included as well, even if you would never choose them in practice. This can help you adopt a flexible approach to the problem.

Try to **think broadly**. Useful questions to help you to think up possible solutions might include:

- What advice would I give a friend who was trying to tackle the same problem? (Sometimes we can think of solutions for others more easily than for ourselves.)
- What ridiculous solutions can I include, as well as more sensible ideas?
- What helpful ideas would others (e.g. family, friends, work colleagues) suggest?
- What approaches have I tried in the past in similar circumstances?

If you feel stuck, sometimes doing this task with someone you trust can be helpful.
Possible options (including ridiculous ideas at first) are:

....

....

....

Step 3: look at the advantages and disadvantages of each possible solution

The next step is to think about the pros and cons of each option you came up with.

My suggestions	Advantages	Disadvantages

Step 4: choose one of the solutions

The chosen solution should be an option that will be a sensible way of tackling your problem. It should be realistic and likely to succeed. The sort of solution you are looking for as a first step is, therefore, something that gets you moving in the right direction. This should be small enough to be possible but big enough to move you forwards. The decision needs to be based on all the answers to Step 3.

Write your preferred solution here:

✎

....

....

....

The solution should be an option that fulfils the following criteria:

Will it be **useful** for changing how you are?	Yes ☐	No ☐
Is it a **clear** task, so that you will know when you have done it?	Yes ☐	No ☐
Is it **realistic**, practical and achievable?	Yes ☐	No ☐

Step 5: plan the steps needed to carry it out

Write down the practical steps needed to carry out your plan. Try to be very specific in your plan so that you know **what** you are going to do and **when** you are going to do it. Include ways of tackling any possible blocks that might get in the way:

✎

....

....

....

....

....

....

Your task is to carry this out during the next week.

Next, check your plan against each of the questions for effective change. Is my planned task one that:

Will be useful for understanding or changing how I am?	Yes ☐	No ☐
Is specific, so that I will know when I have done it?	Yes ☐	No ☐
Is realistic, practical and achievable?	Yes ☐	No ☐
Makes clear what I am going to do and when I am going to do it?	Yes ☐	No ☐
Is an activity that won't be easily blocked or prevented by practical problems?	Yes ☐	No ☐
Will help me to learn useful things, even if it doesn't work out perfectly?	Yes ☐	No ☐

You should be able to answer yes to each of these questions. If your current plan has failed on one of the questions, try to change things so that any poorly planned aspects are improved.

Many people find this approach takes quite a lot of practice. It may also be tempting to be too ambitious. Before moving on, ask yourself again whether this is a target activity that you can cope with at present. If not, swap it for a smaller, more realistic target. Remember that large changes can be achieved by moving one step at a time. Do not push yourself too hard by being overly ambitious.

(!) IMPORTANT POINT

Part of this planning phase should include planning what you will do if your initial plan doesn't work out fully. What if it doesn't work out? Write your plan here:

....

....

....

Step 6: carry out the plan

Carry out your plan and pay attention to your thoughts about what will happen before, during and after you have completed the activity.

Step 7: review the outcome

Write what happened here:

....

....

....

Was the approach successful?	Yes ☐	No ☐
Did it help improve things?	Yes ☐	No ☐
Were there any disadvantages to using this approach?	Yes ☐	No ☐

(?) What have you learned from doing this? Write down any helpful lessons or information you have learned from what happened. If things didn't go quite as you hoped, try to learn from this. How could you make things different during your next attempt to tackle the problem?

....

....

....

If you noticed problems with your plan

Choosing realistic targets for change is important. Were you too ambitious or unrealistic in choosing the target you did? Sometimes a problem-solving approach may be blocked when something happens unexpectedly. Perhaps something didn't happen as you planned, or someone reacted in an unexpected way? Try to learn from what happened.

(?) How could you change how you approach the problem and continue to apply the questions for effective change to help you create a realistic action plan?

....

....

....

Section 4   Planning the next steps

Now that you have considered how your first planned target went, the next step is to plan another change to build on this. You need to think about your **short-, medium-** and **longer-term** targets. Did your plan help you to resolve the problem completely? You may need to plan out other solutions in order to tackle different aspects of your unhelpful behaviour.

You will need to build slowly on what you have done in a step-by-step way. This can be done in the same way that Paul reduced his drinking gradually.

You have the choice to:
- Stick at the target you have achieved.
- Focus on the same unhelpful behaviour but plan to reduce it further.
- Or select a new unhelpful behaviour to work on.

Each of these choices has advantages and disadvantages. Think about what the advantages and disadvantages may be for you.

Choosing a new unhelpful behaviour to reduce

In order to create a clear plan, the key is to again create your own clear **action plan**. This will help you to practise and reinforce your skills in creating a plan.

Do:
- Plan to alter **only one or two** key unhelpful behaviours over the next week.
- Produce an **action plan** to slowly alter what you do in an effective and planned way.
- Ask yourself the questions for effective change to check that the change is well planned.
- Write down your action plan in detail, so that you will be able to put it into practice this week.

Don't:
- Try to start to alter too many things all at once.
- Choose something that is too ambitious a target to start with.
- Be very negative and think 'Nothing can be done. What's the point? It's a waste of time.' (Instead, try to experiment to find out whether this negative thinking is wholly accurate or helpful.)

Write your action plan here:

....

....

....

....

....

....

....

Plan **what** you will do and **when** you will do it. Learn from what happens so that you can keep putting into practice what you have learned. By doing this, you will be able to bring about slow, steady changes in a planned, step-by-step way. You will be able to slowly rebuild your confidence and increase your control over any unhelpful behaviours.

Workbook summary

In this workbook you have:
- Learned about helpful and unhelpful ways of responding to symptoms.
- Discovered key information about the vicious circle of unhelpful behaviours.
- Learned some brief hints and tips of ways to reduce unhelpful behaviours.
- Practised a structured approach to plan a reduction in an unhelpful behaviour.

Putting into practice what you have learned

Continue to put into practice what you have learned over the next few weeks. Do not try to solve every problem you face all at once, but plan out what to do at a pace that is right for you. Build changes one step at a time.

Acknowledgements

I wish to thank all those who have commented upon this workbook, especially Vicki Coletta and Catriona Kent.

My notes

✎

....

....

....

....

....

....

....

....

....

....

....

....

....

....

....

....

....

....

....

....

....

....

....

....

....

....

....

My notes

✎

....

My unhelpful behaviour diary

Day and date	Morning	Afternoon	Evening	Total time spent (or units drunk for alcohol) per day
Monday				
Tuesday				
Wednesday				
Thursday				
Friday				
Saturday				
Sunday				
			Weekly total =	

Remember to record every time you do the unhelpful behaviour.

A Five Areas Approach © Dr C J Williams (2006)

Alcohol, drugs and you

Dr Chris Williams

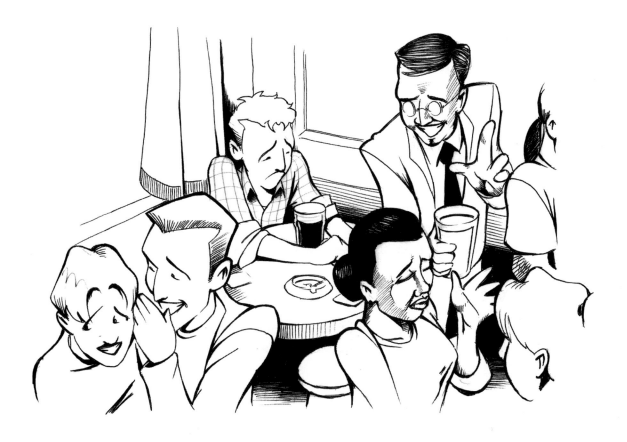

A Five Areas Approach
Helping you to help yourself
www.livinglifetothefull.com

Introduction

Alcohol and street drugs are widely used socially – for fun, for relaxation and for enjoyment. However, they can both be misused and street drugs are illegal.

Using alcohol

Surveys show that many people develop drink problems. People may start drinking to fit in with the crowd, to enjoy the impact of drink, or to block out uncomfortable feelings. However, when alcohol is taken at a high level for weeks or months it can affect our mood, our bodies and our relationships.

 KEY POINT

The recommended highest levels of alcohol to be taken each week are:
- 22 units for women and
- 28 units for men.

1 unit is generally half a pint of bitter or lager, or 1 glass of wine, or one measure of spirits. These values vary, so stronger lagers or beers, or fortified wines etc. will contain far more than one unit of alcohol. Look at the back of the bottle which will say how many units of alcohol are held in standard size glasses.

Using street drugs

People use street drugs for similar reasons to alcohol. A wide range of street drugs exist and even when one type is bought, street samples may be contaminated with all sorts of other things. While the effects of different drugs vary, there are some general effects that they and alcohol can all have.

For more information about street drugs, see www.talktofrank.com.

Recording what you drink and what drugs you use

Everybody is different. Whether you are drinking or taking street drugs a good first step is to record how much you use. Most people underestimate how much they take.

(?) How many units of alcohol do you drink:
A day (what, how much and how many times) ....
A week (what, how much and how many times) ....
How many units is that a week? .... units
How much are you spending a week? £ ....

(?) What street drugs are you taking:
A day (what, how much and how many times) ....
A week (what, how much and how many times) ....
How much are you spending a week? £....................

In answering this question, it is important to bear in mind that we all have a tendency to underestimate our drinking. For example, if like me you have some extra-large wine glasses, then these are not the same as one unit. Some can hold half a bottle of wine, so ten glasses a week (which sounds fine) is actually 5 bottles of wine (which isn't).

The best way of finding out how much you drink in a week is to keep a **diary**. You can find one at the back of this workbook. Try to fill it in each and every time you drink or use drugs. At the end of the week add up the units.

The impact of alcohol on you

Alcohol and drugs, when taken at high levels – or regularly at low levels – can cause a range of problems. Think about the following questions.

Thinking/psychological changes as a result of alcohol/drugs:

People often drink or use drugs to improve how they feel. But they can cause low mood and prevent recovery from depression.

They can:

- Worsen worry and panic attacks.
- Lead to acute bouts of confusion or violence in drunkenness.
- Damage concentration and memory so that it is difficult to learn and retain new information.
- Cause the person to become increasingly suspicious and paranoid.
- Lead to psychological addiction with craving if abruptly stopped.
- Result in irritability and subtle personality changes such as apathy, withdrawal and suspiciousness, which the person may not notice but which will influence their life.

(?) Do you have any of these mental health symptoms?
(Hint: you may need to ask people around you)   Yes ☐   No ☐   Sometimes ☐

Physical changes as a result of alcohol/drugs:

- With drink, the most common symptom is a hangover, with sickness, headaches and dehydration.
- Both alcohol and drugs can lead to physical addiction, with *withdrawal symptoms* such as sweatiness and sickness if abruptly stopped. In severe cases this can lead to alcohol/drug dependency. 'Mental dependency' can also occur even with so-called 'soft' drugs such as cannabis.
- If someone drinks or uses drugs at a high level for some time and suddenly stops drinking (e.g. after admission to hospital) there is a high risk of serious withdrawal that can sometimes be life-threatening. This medically serious condition causes confusion, hallucinations and severe agitation.
- Alcohol can cause damage to parts of the body (for example, stomach ulcers, cirrhosis of the liver, epileptic fits or damage to important body organs such as the pancreas). Drugs can cause lung cancer, heart problems, strokes, fits, can upset body temperature regulation, cause acute confusion, or even sudden death, as they are toxic to many body organs.
- Both alcohol and drug abuse can reduce our ability to fight off infections or serious disease.

(?) Do you have any of these physical symptoms?   Yes ☐   No ☐   Sometimes ☐

Social changes as a result of alcohol/drugs:

- Can cause problems at home, such as arguments with family and friends.
- Often results in debts.
- Can lead to mistakes at work, arriving late, etc. that can cause difficulties, suspensions and loss of job. If you are in education it can cause you difficulties at school, university or college.
- Accidents, violence and car crashes are all common social consequences of alcohol dependency and drug use.

(?) Do you have any of these social symptoms?   Yes ☐   No ☐   Sometimes ☐

(?) Based on your answers to all these questions, overall, do you believe that you are experiencing drink/drug problems?   Yes ☐   No ☐   Sometimes ☐

(!) IMPORTANT POINT

If you are drinking or using drugs in ways that damage you, unless you can reduce the amount you take, you are likely to cause yourself increasing problems in each of these areas. You need to tackle your problem **now**. You may be tempted to downplay or ignore things and believe it is not a problem. Ignoring things is often part of the problem.

EXAMPLE

Paul's drinking

Paul has been off work for a number of months and has developed money worries. He is also concerned about whether he will ever get back to work. He has started to drink more to try and cope. This is now affecting both him and his partner. Look at how this is affecting him.

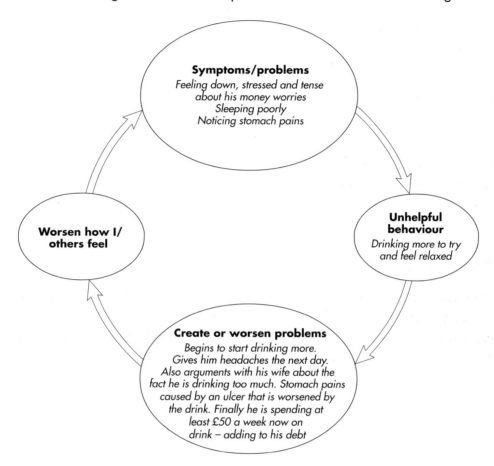

Paul does not actually think he has a drink problem. Instead he sees drink as something that is helpful. This is because he hasn't worked out the unhelpful impact it has on him. He needs to start looking at the downsides of the behaviours as well as the immediate benefits. This means looking at the short and longer term consequences for him and others of his daily drinking.

What impact does his drinking have on Paul and his wife?

Short-term:

● **Physically:** headaches, feel hungover the next day. Stomach pains which are quite bad.

● **Psychologically:** helps me sleep at night to begin with. Makes me feel more relaxed. But then I wake up and have to go to the loo.

● **Socially:** makes me more likely to swear at my wife Sally when she says she is worried about my drinking.

Longer-term (just one year later)

● **Physically:** the stomach ulcer bursts and Paul is admitted to hospital, needing an emergency operation.

● **Psychologically:** alcohol can work as a chemical depressant. It causes anxiety and lowers mood. Paul has become increasingly anxious, angry and depressed.

● **Socially:** Paul tries to return to work but his boss realises he is drinking too much and not coping. He loses his job. Sally cannot cope with how Paul is. They have more and more arguments. Finally she leaves.

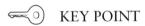 KEY POINT

The difference between *helpful* and *unhelpful* behaviour is that both are done because in the short term they make us feel better. The key difference is that in the longer term our unhelpful behaviours backfire. They worsen how we or others feel. They become part of the problem. The good news is that if this applies to you, you can make changes.

Think about your own drinking. What impact does this have on you and those around you in the short and longer-term?

(?) What impact does the drinking/drug use have on me and those around me?

Short-term:
Physically:

....

....

....

Psychologically:

....

....

....

Socially (on you and others):

....

....

....

And in the **longer-term** (look back over the last 6–12 months)?
Physically:

....

....

....

Psychologically:

....

....

....

Socially (on you and others):

....

....

....

If you have discovered that your drinking/drug use is causing harm to you or others, then you need to tackle it.

Making changes

Try to reduce your overall intake each week. Build in at least **two days** without any drink/drugs to allow your body to recover. You will find the separate workbook *Helpful and unhelpful behaviours* can help you with this.

If you are drinking or using street drugs at a high level

If you stop drinking or taking the drugs too quickly, it is possible you will notice some symptoms of withdrawal. This may be the reason why so many people fail to tackle their problems. However, it is possible to make changes – and, in fact, it is even more important to do so if you are taking drink/drugs at these higher levels.

To make successful changes, you need to cut down the amount taken in a slow step-by-step manner. Again you may find the *Helpful and unhelpful behaviours* workbook helpful. However, for these higher levels of drinking it is best to make changes together with the help and advice of your doctor, local drug/alcohol support services or healthcare practitioner.

(!) IMPORTANT POINT

If you are regularly using street drugs or drinking excessive alcohol, please can you discuss this with someone who can help. If you are doing this on a regular basis, this may act to prevent you getting better.

Extra resources

Look at your Yellow Pages to identify local support services. In addition, ask your doctor. Links to alcohol services are also included at www.livinglifetothefull.com.

My notes

....
....
....
....
....
....
....
....
....
....
....
....
....
....
....
....
....
....
....
....
....
....
....
....
....
....
....

My notes

....

Drink/street drug diary: my week

Day and date	Morning	Afternoon	Evening	Total units per day
Monday				
Tuesday				
Wednesday				
Thursday				
Friday				
Saturday				
Sunday				
				Weekly total =

Remember to record everything you drink/take.

Overcoming sleep problems

Dr Chris Williams

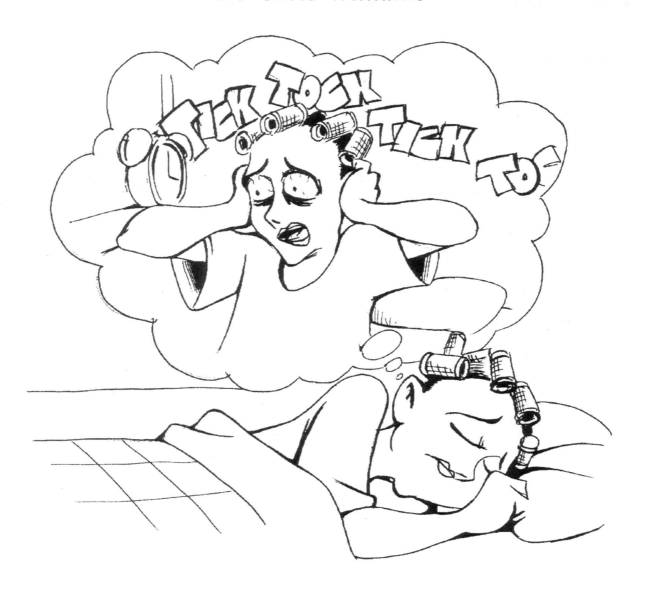

A Five Areas Approach
Helping you to help yourself
www.livinglifetothefull.com

Section 1   Introduction

In this workbook you will learn:
- About sleep and sleeplessness.
- Some common causes of sleep problems.
- How to record your sleep pattern and identify things that worsen your sleep.
- The golden rule for overcoming poor sleep.
- Some other effective changes that will make a difference.
- Hints and tips for overcoming common physical problems.

What is sleep?

Sleep problems are common and affect many people. There is a wide normal healthy sleep range. Some people sleep for only four to six hours a day, whereas others can sleep for as many as 10 or 12 hours a day. Both extremes are quite normal. The amount of sleep each individual needs varies throughout life. Babies and young children need a lot more sleep than older adults. By the time they reach their 60s or 70s, many people find that the amount of sleep they need has dropped by up to several hours a night.

What is insomnia/sleeplessness?

Insomnia is an inability to sleep. Many people have problems sleeping from time to time. Insomnia often starts after an upsetting life event or is caused by a person's lifestyle. A number of different psychological problems can also upset sleep, including anxiety, depression, anger, guilt, shame, and stress at work or in relationships. For example, a person who experiences depression may find that it takes them up to several hours to get off to sleep. They may then wake up several hours earlier than normal, feeling unrested or on edge.

A five areas assessment of sleeplessness

The following factors can worsen sleep. Think about whether they affect your own life.

Area 1: situation, relationship and practical problems

Physical environment: is your bed comfortable? What about the temperature of the room where you sleep? If the room is either very cold or very hot, this might make sleeping difficult. Is the room very noisy? Is there too much light to sleep? If bright lights such as streetlights come through your curtains, this can also prevent sleep.

 Do I try to sleep in a poor sleep environment?   Yes ☐   No ☐

   If yes, the following are some specific things that you can do:
- **Poor mattress:** if your mattress is old, try turning it over, rotating it or changing it. Try adding extra support such as a board or an old door underneath.

- **Too hot/too cold:** if it is too hot, open a window or use a fan. If it is too cold, think about insulation, draught excluders, secondary or double-glazing, etc., or add an extra blanket or duvet.
- **Problems with noise:** reduce noise if you can. Ask noisy neighbours to turn down their television or music. Have you thought about fitting double-glazing or internal plastic sheeting over windows to reduce noise? This need not be expensive: ask your local DIY store about cost-effective alternative options.
- **Problems with excessive light:** consider changing your curtains. Add a thicker lining or blackout lining. If cost is a problem, then a black plastic bin bag can be an effective blackout blind. Staple or stick it to the curtain rail.

Area 2: altered thinking

Anxious thoughts are a common cause of sleeplessness. Anxious thoughts may be about worries in general, or they may focus on worrying about not sleeping. You may worry that it will not be possible to sleep at all or that sleeplessness will reduce your ability to be effective at work. These unrealistic fears prevent you getting off to sleep. Other common fears include worries that your brain or body will be harmed by lack of sleep.

In sleep, there is a reduction in tension levels, leading your body and brain to relax and drop off to sleep. In contrast, in anxiety, the brain becomes overly alert. You end up mulling things over again and again. This is the exact opposite of what is needed to get off to sleep. Worrying thoughts are therefore both a cause and an effect of poor sleep.

(?) Do I worry about things in general?　　　　　　　Yes ☐　　No ☐　　Sometimes ☐

If yes, read the workbook *Noticing and changing extreme and unhelpful thinking.*

(?) Do I worry about not sleeping?　　　　　　　　　Yes ☐　　No ☐　　Sometimes ☐

If yes, jot down some notes of your worries on a notepad. You will need to challenge any catastrophic fears about the consequences of not sleeping. Studies show that most people do not need very much sleep at all in order to be physically and mentally healthy. In sleep research laboratories, it has been found that many people who experience insomnia actually sleep far more than they think. Sometimes people who are in a light level of sleep dream that they are awake. Therefore, you may be sleeping more than you think. You also need to know that sleep deprivation does not have a catastrophic impact on your brain or body. It is possible to function effectively with very little sleep each night.

(?) Do I have extreme or catastrophic fears about the consequences of not sleeping?　　　　　　　　Yes ☐　　No ☐　　Sometimes ☐

Extreme and catastrophic fears can cause increased wakefulness, thus preventing you from getting off to sleep. Being aware that these thoughts are extreme, inaccurate and unhelpful is important. Although you might feel tired and irritable, this does not necessarily affect your ability to perform tasks around the house or at work.

(task) If worrying thoughts are a problem for you, read the workbook *Noticing and changing extreme and unhelpful thinking.*

Area 3: altered physical problems

Pain, itching and other physical symptoms can cause sleeplessness. Tackling these physical symptoms will help sleep problems.

(?) Are physical symptoms keeping me awake?　　　Yes ☐　　No ☐　　Sometimes ☐

If yes, discuss this with your healthcare practitioner. In particular, if you notice that you feel short of breath when you lie down, please discuss this with your doctor. Sometimes this can mean that a water tablet or diuretic is needed. Sometimes symptoms of depression or anxiety can worsen symptoms such as pain; in this case, treating the low or anxious mood will help reduce the pain.

Area 4: altered emotions/feelings

A range of different emotions can be linked to sleeplessness.

(?) Do I feel anxious when I try to sleep?　　　Yes ☐　　No ☐　　Sometimes ☐

Anxiety is a common cause of sleeplessness. It is often associated with a triggering of the body's fight or flight adrenalin response. This can cause the person to feel fidgety or restless. You may notice physical symptoms such as increased heart rate or breathing rate, churning stomach or tension throughout the body. The anxiety therefore acts to keep you alert. This is the opposite of what you want when you are trying to fall off to sleep. Sometimes we become anxious about sleeping, for example if we have nightmares or wake feeling panicky.

(?) Am I feeling depressed, upset or low in mood and
no longer enjoying things as before?　　　Yes ☐　　No ☐　　Sometimes ☐

If yes, depression is a common cause of sleeplessness. For example, a person who is feeling depressed may find that it takes them up to several hours to get off to sleep. They may wake up several hours earlier than normal, feeling unrested or on edge. Treatment of depression can often be helpful in improving sleep.

Other emotions such as shame, guilt and anger can also be linked to sleeplessness.

Area 5: altered and unhelpful behaviours

Preparing for sleep

The time leading up to sleep is very important. Build in a **wind-down time** in the evening when you are less active. Physical overactivity, such as exercising or eating too much just before bed, can keep you awake. Sometimes people read or watch television while lying in bed. This may help them wind down, but for many people it can make them become more alert and add to their sleep problems.

(?) Am I engaging in activities that wake me up when I
should be winding down?　　　Yes ☐　　No ☐　　Sometimes ☐

If yes, keep your bed as a place for sleep and sex. Don't lie on your bed reading, watching TV, working or worrying. This will only wake you up and prevent you sleeping. You need to decide whether listening to the radio or music helps you sleep. Don't exercise in the half-hour before going to sleep, as it may wake you up.

What about caffeine?

Caffeine is a chemical found in coffee, tea, cola drinks, hot chocolate and some herbal drinks. It causes increased alertness. If taken at high levels for several weeks, it can cause physical and psychological addiction. Drinking as few as five strong cups of coffee a day on a regular basis is physically addictive. It also reduces sleep quality. There is a real risk that a vicious circle can occur, whereby tiredness causes the person to drink more coffee to keep alert. Then the coffee itself affects the person's sleep and worsens the original tiredness.

It is important to know that caffeine stays in our bodies for a few hours before it is broken down or leaves in our urine. This means that we should avoid drinking caffeine drinks in the few hours leading up to going to bed.

(?) Am I taking in too much caffeine? Yes ☐ No ☐ Sometimes ☐

If yes, caffeine-containing drinks should be reduced if you are drinking them to excess. If you regularly drink more than five cups of strong coffee a day, try to reduce your total caffeine intake. Do this in a step-by-step way or switch slowly to decaffeinated coffees, cola or teas. Avoid having a cup of coffee or a last cigarette before sleep. Both caffeine and nicotine will keep you awake. Some people find that a warm milky drink helps them get off to sleep.

What about alcohol?

Sometimes people drink alcohol to reduce feelings of tension and help them get off to sleep. One unit of alcohol is about half a pint of beer, one short, or one glass of wine. If you drink more than the recommended level of alcohol (22 units a week for women, 28 units a week for men), then this can cause problems such as anxiety, depression and sleeplessness. Finally, drinking too much alcohol will cause you to go to the toilet more than usual at night. This will keep you awake.

(?) Am I drinking too much alcohol? Yes ☐ No ☐ Sometimes ☐

If yes, getting up in the night to use the toilet can be avoided by reducing the amount you drink before going to bed. If you take a diuretic (a water tablet), you should aim to take it earlier in the day. Discuss this with your doctor. If you drink more than the healthy amount of alcohol, try to cut down the amount in a slow step-by-step manner. Discuss how best to do this with your healthcare practitioner or read the workbook *Helpful and unhelpful things we can do*.

What about your sleep pattern?

If you are not sleeping well, it can be tempting to go to bed either very much earlier or very much later than normal. Napping is another habit that can end up backfiring by upsetting the natural sleep–wake cycle. Try to get up before 9 a.m. unless you are on shift work, which makes this impractical.

(?) Do I have a disrupted sleep pattern (going to bed/getting up)? Yes ☐ No ☐ Sometimes ☐

If yes, set yourself regular sleep times. Get up at a set time, even if you have slept poorly. Try to teach your body what time to fall asleep and what time to get up. Go to sleep some time between 10 p.m. and midnight. Try to get up at a sensible time between 7 a.m. and 9 a.m. Adjust these times to fit your own circumstances.

Tossing and turning in bed and clock-watching

 Do you find yourself lying awake in bed tossing and turning, waking your partner up to talk ('Are you awake?') or just watching the clock? Yes ☐ No ☐ Sometimes ☐

 KEY POINT

If you cannot sleep, get up out of bed if you are not sleeping after 20 minutes. Go downstairs and do something else until you are 'sleepy tired' again. Then return to bed. Do this again and again until you go to sleep. When downstairs, don't do things that will make you more active, e.g. watching a scary film.

This idea of getting up if you aren't sleeping is such an important principle that it is sometimes called 'the golden rule'.

Recording your sleep

You may find it helpful to use a **sleep diary** for a few days this week as you use this workbook. A blank sleep diary is included at the end of this workbook. Copy out the headings or photocopy it. By completing the diary, you will identify important factors that affect your sleep.

Carrying out your own five areas assessment

(task) Look at the five areas assessment diagram below. Write in all the factors you have identified that affect you. These are possible targets for change.

Five areas assessment of factors affecting my own sleep

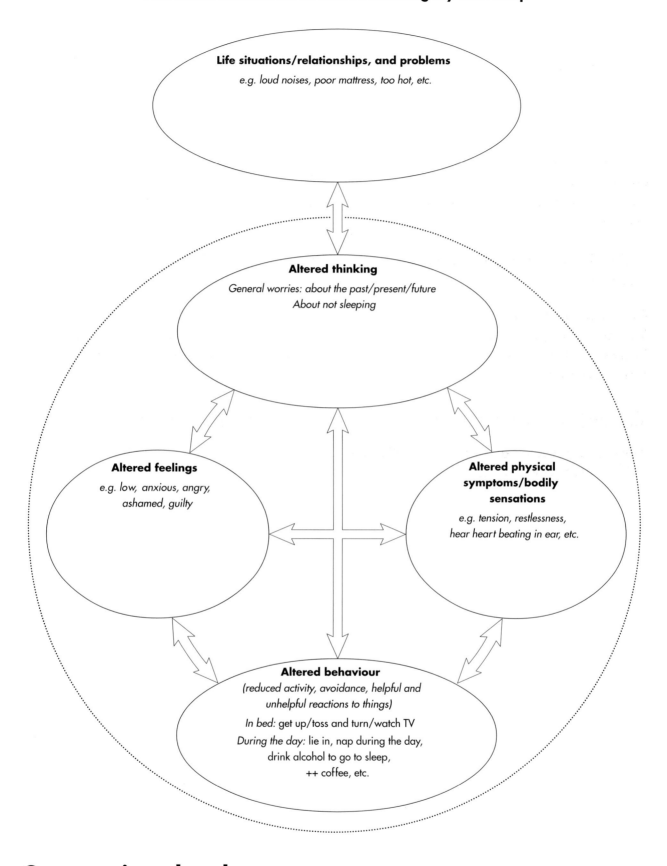

Overcoming sleeplessness

 My sleep checklist: some things to do and not do

Use the checklists below to find out about things you can do to overcome your own sleep problems:

Some things to do in the run-up to bed and during the day	Tick here if this affects your own life, even if only sometimes	Some changes you can make/resources to use
Live by the golden rule: bed is only for sleep and sex		Get up out of bed if you are not sleeping after 20 minutes. Go downstairs and do something else until you are 'sleepy tired' again. Then return to bed. Do this again and again until you go to sleep. When downstairs, don't do things that will make you more active
Adopt a regular time to go to bed and to get up		See earlier in this workbook
Tackle things you know affect your sleep environment, e.g. noise, mattress, etc.		See earlier in this workbook. If neighbours cause noise, read the workbooks *Practical problem-solving* and *Being assertive*. Consider the surroundings (noise, light levels, temperature, comfort of your bed). Plan changes to your room, mattress, etc. as needed.
Reduce your general life pressures		Say no. Balance demands you put on yourself. Allow space and time for you
Plan a wind-down time each evening		See earlier in this workbook. Warm bran-based milky drinks may help. Consider having a bath and listening to relaxing music. If you like them, consider using candles, scented oils, etc.
Stop, think and reflect on worrying thoughts about the past/present/future and also about sleep		If worrying thoughts keep you awake, get up and go downstairs (the golden rule). When downstairs **write down the worries**. Decide to worry or think about them tomorrow during the day.[1] Use the workbook *Noticing and changing extreme and unhelpful thinking* to put the thoughts into perspective next day
Live reasonably healthily: fitter people generally sleep better		Strange as it sounds, overdoing healthy living may become unhealthy, e.g. overexercising. Try to live healthily but not obsessively so
Use relaxation tapes/techniques if you find them helpful		Free downloadable/streaming relaxation resources using anxiety-control training (originally developed by Dr Philip Snaith) are available. See our support site for this book at www.livinglifetothefull.com
If you are prescribed tablets such as antidepressant medication, take them regularly		If you are taking diuretics or water tablets, then consider whether they are making you wake at night to go to the toilet. It may be possible to change the time of day these are taken. Discuss any changes with your doctor

[1]This approach was originally developed by Dr Tom Borkevic, who advises that you use a diary list of worries. Write them down and then plan a specific 'worry time' the following day. Many people find that the worries fade significantly in the cool light of day.

Some things not to do in the run up to bed and during the day	Tick here if this affects your own life, even if only sometimes	Some changes you can make/resources to use
Drinking too much alcohol or caffeine or smoking too much		See earlier in this workbook. Alcohol causes sleep to be shallow and unrefreshing. It can also make you wake up more to use the toilet. Don't drink too much coffee, tea, hot chocolate or cola drinks, which contain caffeine. Around five cups or glasses a day of caffeine-containing drinks should be the maximum. Switch to decaffeinated drinks or water beyond this. Nicotine in cigarettes causes sleeplessness. Don't smoke just before bed. Medical treatments such as nicotine patches may help you to reduce or stop smoking
Doing things that stimulate you mentally or physically in the run-up to sleep e.g. working or doing crosswords		You can of course do these things, but plan to stop doing them in the last hour or so before going to bed. Avoid doing puzzles, reading, watching television, etc. in bed (see the golden rule)
Letting problems build up unaddressed, so you worry about them at night		Again, note them down and deal with them tomorrow
Responding in ways that end up backfiring or worsening things, e.g. lying in during the day or napping		Make efforts to reset your body clock by getting up at a set time each day. Avoid napping and plan to go to bed at roughly the same time each day
Looking for an answer to sleeplessness in sleeping tablets		Sleeping tablets are not a long-term solution, and many can cause problems of addiction. See the workbook *Understanding and using antidepressant medication*, which includes a short section on minor tranquillisers and sleeping tablets

Don't expect to change everything immediately. With practice, however, you can make helpful changes to your sleep pattern. If you have difficulties, just do what you can.

Your five areas assessment should have helped you identify the problems you currently face. The table above should have provided you with hints and tips on each of the main problem areas.

 CHOICE POINT

The next section of this workbook briefly covers how low mood and depression can affect our body. You may wish to complete this. If not, skip to Section 3.

Section 2 Hints and tips for overcoming common physical changes in low mood and anxiety

The following is a short practical summary of some immediate changes that you can bring about that may help some of the physical symptoms you are experiencing.

Physical symptoms of depression and anxiety	Hints and tips
Difficulties getting off to sleep	Try to get into a routine: go to bed and get up at a regular time
	Avoid napping during the day: it upsets your body clock
	Avoid drinking too much coffee, tea, hot chocolate and soft drinks, which contain caffeine: around five cups or glasses a day is the maximum. Switch to decaffeinated drinks if you drink more than this
	Watch your alcohol intake: alcohol causes sleep to be shallow and unrefreshing
Wakening earlier than usual	This is common in depression and improves as the depression lifts
	Try to rest in bed
	If you feel agitated, get up. Consider medication to reduce agitation if this is a problem; discuss this with your doctor
	Try to get up before 9 a.m. each day
	Lying in or napping during the day is likely to upset your body clock and add to your problems
Disrupted sleep pattern	Sleep problems are common in depression and anxiety. They will not cause any immediate harm to your body or your mind
	If you find yourself waking up repeatedly during the night, get up, do something else (e.g. read or watch television, but avoid scary films, which may wake you up still further) until you feel 'sleepy tired', then go to bed again. It is important not to sleep or nap during the next day, even if you feel tired
Decreased appetite	Eating a balanced range of foods is important to keep up both your physical and your mental strength
	Try to eat foods that contain energy, such as protein, fats and carbohydrate, and also fruit and vegetables
Increased appetite	Try to eat a balanced and sensible diet
	Plan your shopping to avoid impulse buys, particularly of carbohydrates such as biscuits and chocolate ('comfort eating' may occur)
	Try to avoid increasing your alcohol intake, which may worsen your depression or anxiety

Physical symptoms of depression and anxiety	Hints and tips
Increased appetite	Try to eat meals at a dining table. Avoid snacking or bringing extra food to the table. If you want to eat more, force yourself to get up, so that it is a conscious decision to eat it
Weight	Reduced activity levels and increased appetite may cause weight gain. Think about introducing some mild exercise into your day (this may also boost your mood)
	Eat a balanced diet: vegetables and fruit will also prevent constipation
Decreased weight	Eating a balanced range of foods is important to keep up both your physical and your mental strength
	Try to keep eating a balanced range of foods that contain energy, such as protein, fats and carbohydrate, and also fruit and vegetables
Reduced energy	Low energy is a common problem in depression
	A vicious circle can arise. By reducing your activity, you use your muscles less. This causes them to weaken and feel painful and tired when you do use them
	An effective way of overcoming this is to plan a graded increase in your activity in a step-by-step way
	This often leads to a boost in how you feel mentally as well as physically
	Remember: don't overdo exercise. Plan a slow increase in what you do. Just five minutes of exercise, e.g. walking up and down the stairs three times a day to begin with, is the sort of level to aim at if you have not been doing any exercise recently. Slowly increase this over the next few days and weeks
	If you have a physical illness, discuss exercise with your doctor and agree a plan for this graded increase in activity that is appropriate for you
	A common symptom in depression is to feel worse first thing in the morning. If you notice this, plan to do activities and go out later on in the day
	Don't throw yourself into this too quickly. Do it one step at a time. See the workbook *Overcoming reduced activity and avoidance*
Reduced sex drive	Reduced sex drive is common in depression and anxiety. If you have a partner, try to discuss this with them
	Your sex drive will improve (as will other symptoms) towards its previous levels as you recover from low or anxious mood
	In men, antidepressants sometimes cause problems with erections and ejaculation. In women, antidepressants sometimes reduce or prevent the experience of orgasm. If this is a difficulty for you and you are taking antidepressants, discuss this with your doctor

Physical symptoms of depression and anxiety	Hints and tips
Reduced sex drive	If you find it difficult talking about your sexual problems with your partner, try to discuss the problems with your healthcare practitioner
Symptoms of constipation	Constipation commonly occurs in depression. Simple changes can help
	Eat vegetables, bran and fibre
	Exercise can help
	Drink a reasonable amount of fluids
	Constipation can be a side effect of some antidepressants
Symptoms of pain	Chest pain, stomach pain and headaches may be worsened by depression or anxiety. If this is the case for you, treating the depression or anxiety can be an effective pain reliever
	If the pain is linked to the depression or anxiety, you may find that painkillers such as aspirin and paracetamol do not seem to be very effective
	If this is the case, it is important to avoid building up the dose of painkillers you are taking, as this may cause new physical symptoms; for some people, painkillers may even cause more symptoms of pain and possibly addiction
	In this case, treatment with antidepressants is often more effective. Discuss this with your doctor. Also discuss with your doctor how to reduce slowly any painkillers that are no longer needed
Symptoms of physical agitation	Focusing your attention on these symptoms can sometimes worsen them. This mental tension then adds to the unpleasant physical tension feelings
	If the agitation feelings are very distressing, consider using medication to reduce them. Many effective short-term medications (which are not addictive) are available. In addition, antidepressant medication will often improve symptoms of agitation caused by depression
	Note that some symptoms of agitation can be caused by antidepressant medications. If agitation rises significantly shortly after starting or increasing the dose of an antidepressant, discuss this with your doctor

Section 3   **Summary**

In this workbook you have learned:
- About sleep and sleeplessness.
- Some common causes of sleep problems.
- How to record your sleep pattern and identify things that worsen your sleep.
- The golden rule for overcoming poor sleep.
- Some other effective changes that will make a difference.
- Hints and tips for overcoming common physical problems.

Putting into practice what you have learned

Look back at the sleep checklists of things to do and not do on pages 8–9. Plan to make changes in how you prepare for sleep and what you do once you are in bed. The single most effective thing you can do to improve your sleep is to **follow the golden rule**.

Write down what you are going to do this week to put into practice what you have learned.

(?) What changes am I going to make?

✎
....
....
....

(?) When am I going to do it?

✎
....
....
....

(?) What problems/difficulties could arise, and how can I overcome these?

✎
....
....
....

Apply the questions for effective change to your plan. Is my planned task one that:

Will be useful for understanding or changing how I am?	Yes ☐	No ☐
Is a specific task, so that I will know when I have done it?	Yes ☐	No ☐
Is realistic, practical and achievable?	Yes ☐	No ☐
Makes clear what I am going to do and when I am going to do it?	Yes ☐	No ☐
Is an activity that won't be easily blocked or prevented by practical problems?	Yes ☐	No ☐
Will help me to learn useful things even if it doesn't work out perfectly?	Yes ☐	No ☐

Remember to review your progress in making these changes on a weekly basis and to make sure the changes are practical and achievable.

Acknowledgements

I wish to thank all those who have commented upon this workbook, especially Marie Chellingsworth and Dr Frances Cole.

My notes

....

....

....

....

....

....

....

....

....

....

....

....

....

....

....

....

....

....

....

....

....

....

....

....

....

....

....

....

My notes

....

My sleep diary

Time when you are in bed/ trying to sleep	Record when you are asleep with a X	When in bed, record any thoughts/images that go through your mind and keep you awake (e.g. worries, fears about sleeping/ consequences of not sleeping)	Record any activities you do that relate to sleep before bed (e.g. alcohol, caffeine, smoking, exercise, daytime napping, sleeping in) and in bed (e.g. reading, radio, crosswords, talking to partner, tossing and turning, getting up, going downstairs)
8–9.59 p.m.			
10–11.59 p.m.			
12–1.59 a.m.			
2–3.59 a.m.			
4–5.59 a.m.			
6–7.59 a.m.			
8–9.59 a.m.			
10–11.59 a.m.			
12–1.59 p.m.			
2–3.59 p.m.			
4–5.59 p.m.			
6–7.59 p.m.			

Understanding and using antidepressant medication

Dr Chris Williams

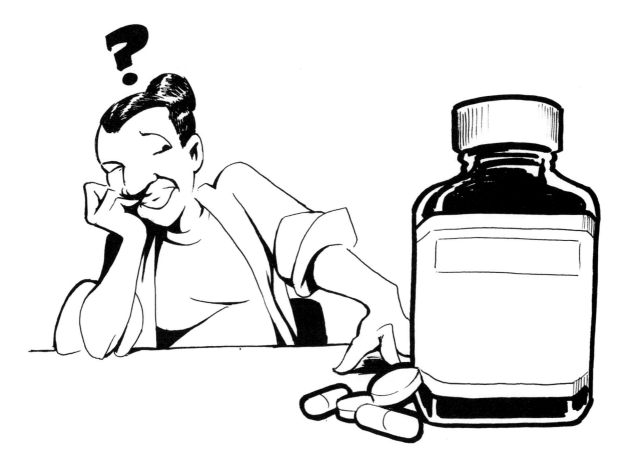

A Five Areas Approach
Helping you to help yourself
www.livinglifetothefull.com

Introduction

This workbook is written for anyone who is taking antidepressant medication or who wishes to find out more about the uses of these types of medicine.

In this workbook you will learn:

- Why antidepressants can be used as a treatment for depression and anxiety.
- About the advantages and disadvantages of using antidepressant medication.
- About your own attitudes towards the use of antidepressants.
- Ways of using any medication more effectively.

No names of any specific medications are mentioned in the workbook. Instead, the aim is to inform you about the general principles of using tablet approaches. You can obtain details of different antidepressant medications from your own doctor or healthcare practitioner.

Introductory information

A large number of different antidepressants exist. They are most often helpful when there is:

- Moderate or severe symptoms of depression, e.g. **low mood and lack of enjoyment.**
- Several of the physical changes of depression, e.g. **low energy, reduced concentration, altered sleep or appetite.**
- Significant agitation or onset or worsening of suspiciousness or panic.
- Suicidal ideas, where you can't see a future.

Antidepressants are not usually helpful for problems of mildly low mood.

Antidepressants are also used to treat a variety of other mental and physical health problems. These include:

- **Generalised anxiety,** where there is anxious worrying about lots of different things. The worry is strong enough to cause physical symptoms of anxiety. It also has an impact on the person's behaviour or activity.
- **Panic attacks** and some **phobic disorders,** where levels of anxiety reach such a high peak that the person fears something terrible will occur. This causes the person to stop what they are doing and hurry away.
- **Obsessive–compulsive disorder** (OCD). Here, the person is plagued by recurrent intrusive thoughts, impulses or images. They find these distressing and try hard to avoid thinking like this. OCD often leads to various actions designed to prevent harm occurring. This includes checking or cleaning things again and again, or doing things in a very repetitive way.
- **Physical symptoms,** such as chronic fatigue and pain.

Key information

Why use antidepressant medications for the treatment of depression?

Links exist between the altered thinking, feelings, behaviour and physical aspects of depression. Look at the arrows in the diagram. Each of these five areas affects the others and offers possible areas of change in order to improve things. Intervention in any one area can lead to improvements in the others.

The five areas assessment model

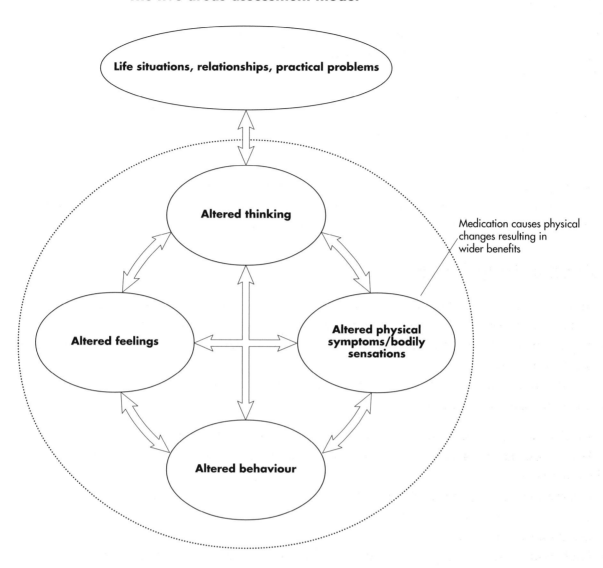

Because of the links between each of the areas, the physical treatment offered by medication can lead to positive improvements in the other areas too. Medication aims to relieve the physical symptoms of depression. In turn, this can help the person feel better and able to work at changing any unhelpful behaviours.

KEY POINT

Antidepressants are the fastest and most effective way of improving your depression in the short term. If you are feeling very depressed, they can help you get to a stage where you are able to manage your symptoms better. They also help prevent relapses and can help you deal with any future episodes so they are not so severe or prolonged. If you are taking an antidepressant, or wish to know whether taking one is likely to be helpful for you, you should discuss this with your doctor. **Please do not stop taking antidepressants without discussing it with your doctor.**

Stopping antidepressants

Sometimes we may be tempted to stop taking medication without telling our doctor. We may be afraid we are letting them down or that we will be told off if we do. It is far better to discuss any concerns you have openly with your doctor. It is also important when stopping antidepressants to do this gradually. Otherwise, symptoms caused by this sudden stopping may sometimes occur (see page 5).

How effective are antidepressant tablets?

Antidepressants can help lift symptoms in moderate or severe depression in approximately two-thirds of people. This figure increases further still when different combinations of medication are used. The best outcomes are usually achieved when psychological approaches such as cognitive behaviour therapy are used at the same time.

How long do they take to work?

Most people notice a substantial improvement in how they feel within two weeks of starting an antidepressant. Antidepressants take about **two weeks to begin to work**, and their positive actions may take up to four to six weeks to reach a peak. It is very important, therefore, to take the tablets regularly and for long enough, even if to begin with it seems as if they are not working. Most antidepressant medications are started at lower doses and may then be slowly increased in dose over a number of weeks or months if this is needed. Therefore it is important to take the tablets regularly and for long enough if prescribed. If there is little or no improvement, then an increase in dose, change of medication and fresh look at other problems may be needed. There are lots of different types of antidepressant, and your doctor may wish to change your medication to ensure the right one is found for you.

 IMPORTANT POINT

A common problem is that a person stops the antidepressants when they first feel well again. Stopping an antidepressant too early is a common cause of worsening depression. It is usually necessary to take the antidepressant medication for at least six months after feeling better to prevent slipping back into depression.

Medication as part of an overall package of care

The treatment package should also include learning new ways of tackling your low mood and distress. Overall, treatment with cognitive behaviour therapy and some other psychological treatments seems to be as effective as antidepressant medication for mild to moderate levels of depression. There are also benefits of using both approaches together. Medication may be especially helpful when low mood or tension makes it difficult for you to achieve change using a psychological approach alone.

 KEY POINT

Benzodiazepines (minor tranquillisers)

Benzodiazepines have been used widely for the treatment of symptoms of anxiety. They are commonly called tranquillisers and are also used as sleeping tablets. It is important to note that although these tablets are sometimes prescribed to treat some of the symptoms of depression, such as sleeplessness, these tablets do not treat depression and are not antidepressants.

Benzodiazepines can, unfortunately, cause new problems if taken for a long time, as higher and higher doses are often required to have the same effect. Because of this need to take more tablets and the occurrence of problems with withdrawal, they may become addictive. They commonly also cause side effects of tiredness and problems with concentration. When benzodiazepines are taken on a regular basis, about one in three people experiences problems of addiction. The risk of addiction is higher if you have had problems of addiction with illegal drugs, other medications or alcohol. If you become addicted to benzodiazepines, suddenly stopping the tablets may lead to problems of worsening tension and distress. There may also be physical symptoms such as feeling sweaty and shaky with a rapid heart and sleeplessness. This can occur up to three weeks or more after stopping the medication. Due to this problem of addiction, doctors prescribe these medicines much less commonly nowadays. The dose should be limited to the lowest possible dose for the shortest possible time. Benzodiazepines are short-term medications and are not usually for long-term use.

If you have been prescribed benzodiazepines for a long time, it is important that any change of medication is done at the right pace and with the agreement of your doctor. Please do not suddenly stop any regular medication without a discussion with them. There are some very effective treatment programmes that can help you reduce and stop long-term benzodiazepine use. These treatments usually combine medication and psychological treatments. If you find yourself in this situation, please discuss it with your doctor or healthcare practitioner.

Do antidepressants have side effects?

All tablets have side effects. The important question is whether the side effects of having untreated depression are worse. Modern antidepressants are often not very sedating and do not cause much weight gain. Many side effects disappear within a few days of starting the tablets as you get used to them. Sometimes anxiety can actually worsen how much we notice symptoms.

If you notice side effects, your doctor may be able to reduce the dose or change the tablet to another one. The key question is whether on balance the antidepressants have helped or hindered you.

If your answer to this is that they have helped, then keep taking them as advised by your doctor. If you feel they have not helped you, then please do not stop them yourself. Instead, discuss this with your doctor. Perhaps the dose of the medication can be altered, or another medication may be more suitable. Whatever your decision, please do not decide to stop taking your medication without discussing it with your doctor.

Can I drive or use machinery if I take tablets?

Many antidepressant medications can affect your ability to drive and operate machinery. They can also exaggerate the effects of alcohol. Read the medication advice leaflet that accompanies your prescription to see whether this applies to you, or ask your doctor or pharmacist if in any doubt.

My attitudes towards medication

Antidepressant medications are sometimes viewed with suspicion. Think about whether any of the following apply to you:

(?) Do I worry that they are addictive?   Yes ☐   No ☐   Sometimes ☐

It is not possible to become addicted to modern antidepressants in the same way as alcohol or other tablets such as benzodiazepines. Antidepressants do need to be taken sensibly and as recommended by your doctor. If tablets are started at too high an initial dose, side effects are more common; similarly, if a tablet taken at a high dose is stopped suddenly, some short-lived **discontinuation symptoms** may occur. To prevent this, many tablets are first started by slowly increasing the dose and then later stopped by tapering down their dose over several days.

(?) Do I think I should get better on my own without
taking tablets?   Yes ☐   No ☐   Sometimes ☐

Antidepressant medications are one of a number of important ways of helping yourself get better. They can helpfully alter some of the physical symptoms that occur in depression as well as boosting how you feel. They do not replace the need for you to work at changing other aspects of your life, such as tackling relationship issues or other practical problems. At the same time, antidepressants taken when needed can be a really important part of your treatment package and can help you make changes that you would otherwise struggle to do. Your body, thoughts and emotional feelings are all part of you – they are not in separate boxes. If you have broken a leg, you are unlikely to say 'I want to get better by myself without medical treatment.' Why do the same in depression? If your doctor is recommending antidepressants, discuss why they suggest this, so that you can jointly make the decision about whether it is the right thing for you at the moment.

(?) Do I ever try to cope without my tablets?[1]   Yes ☐   No ☐   Sometimes ☐

When tablets are prescribed to be taken every day, it is important to do this or it may prevent them from being effective. Many people miss their tablets on occasion (or more often) for a variety of reasons. If you decide that the tablets are not for you, it is best to discuss this with your doctor. Then you can agree jointly on how best to work on your problems.

Practical problems taking medication

Remembering to take the tablets

For almost any medication, it may be difficult to remember to take them on a regular basis. This is particularly the case in depression, because of the poor concentration and forgetfulness that can often occur.

(?) Do I sometimes forget to take my medication?   Yes ☐   No ☐   Sometimes ☐

The following may help you to remember to take your tablets:
- Get into a routine. Take the tablets at a set time each day.
- Place the tablets somewhere where you will see them when you get up or go to bed. For example, place them by your toothbrush. Make sure children can't take them by mistake.
- Write little notes to yourself saying 'medication'. Use coloured pieces of paper to help remind you if you don't want others to read your notes. Place them where you will see them at the time you need to take the tablets. Stick them on the fridge, oven, computer or back door so that you are reminded throughout the day.
- Set an alarm using your watch, an alarm clock or the alarm function on a telephone to remind you to take them at a set time.
- Recruit other people to remind you or telephone you if you find that you struggle to remember otherwise.

Getting into a routine to avoid confusion

(?) Do I ever get confused about whether I have taken
the medication?   Yes ☐   No ☐   Sometimes ☐

[1]Thanks to Dr David Thompson for this useful question.

Antidepressant medication generally needs to be taken regularly in order to be effective. The following can help you to be clear about when you have taken your medication:

- Tick off the doses you have taken in a diary or calendar. You may find that attaching a wallet-sized card calendar to the medication box can be a helpful way to do this. These calendars are usually available free of charge from your local pharmacy.
- A dosette box can help if you are taking lots of tablets at different times each day. These have different compartments for each time of day. You can fill up the box in advance for the whole week. If this is difficult, you could ask a friend, neighbour or healthcare practitioner to help. Dosette boxes are usually available from your pharmacist.

Misusing tablets

 Do I ever take a higher dose than is prescribed?   Yes ☐   No ☐   Sometimes ☐

Medication can be a useful and helpful addition to treatment when low mood is severe or prolonged. However, there are several possible pitfalls in starting or stopping such medication. For example, it can be tempting to take extra tablets at times of higher distress in order to cope, even when the tablets aren't prescribed with this in mind. This forms one of the **unhelpful responses** described in the workbook *Helpful and unhelpful things we do*. Misusing tablets in this way can backfire and worsen the situation because:

- Tablets taken at higher than recommended doses may cause unpleasant side effects or be potentially dangerous.
- It teaches you that you are managing to cope only because of using the higher dose. The danger is that you then come to believe that you need the extra medication and are scared to live life without tablets.

  KEY POINT

It is very important not to take a higher dose of tablets than your doctor prescribes. Most antidepressant tablets usually work over a number of weeks. Taking more on one particular day will have little or no impact on your depression. Tablets taken at higher than recommended doses can cause unpleasant side effects or be dangerous. If you are concerned that your medication is not working, please discuss this with your doctor. Remember that significant improvement with antidepressants often takes place within the first two weeks of taking the tablets. In addition, the benefits tend to continue to build up over the next few weeks after this.

Conclusions

When deciding whether to start or continue an antidepressant, the key question is whether taking the tablets will help you improve how you feel. Regardless of whether you take medications, psychological treatments such as the cognitive behaviour therapy approach used in the *Overcoming Depression and Low Mood* course are an important part of treatment.

- Antidepressants may have an important role in helping people with depression get better.
- Antidepressants are not addictive. However, when stopping higher doses it is sensible to reduce the dose slowly over a period of time to prevent discontinuation symptoms.
- Taking the tablets on a regular basis is essential for them to work.
- All tablets have side effects. However, for most people the benefits of antidepressants far outweigh the costs.

Finding out more

The website run by the British Pharmacological Society provides a central page that links to sites summarising this information. See www.bps.ac.uk/link/linkdruginfo.jsp.

Workbook summary

In this workbook, you have learned:
- Why antidepressants can be used as a treatment for depression and anxiety.
- The advantages and disadvantages of using antidepressant medication.
- Your own attitudes towards the use of antidepressants.
- Ways of using any medication more effectively.

Putting into practice what you have learned

If you want to find out more about the use of antidepressant medications, please discuss this with your doctor, healthcare practitioner or pharmacist. They will be able to suggest other sources of information about the treatments that are available.

Acknowledgements

I wish to thank all those who have commented upon this workbook, especially Dr Joe Bouch, Marie Chellingsworth, Celia Scott-Warren and Dr Stephen Williams.

My notes

....

....

....

....

....

....

....

....

....

....

....

....

....

....

....

....

....

....

....

....

....

....

....

....

....

....

....

Planning for the future

Dr Chris Williams

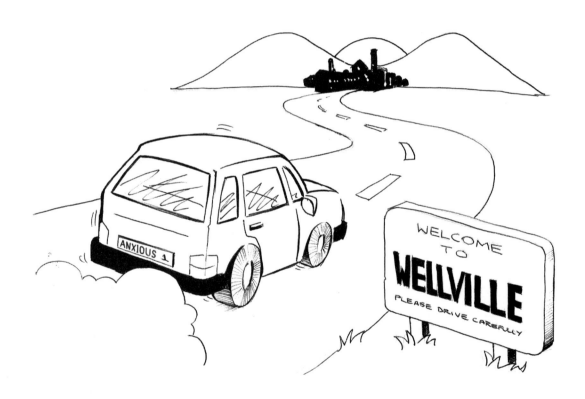

A Five Areas Approach
Helping you to help yourself
www.livinglifetothefull.com

Section 1   Introduction

In this workbook you will:

- Summarise what you have learned about getting better.
- Create a mental fitness plan to use in the future.
- Produce a list of your own **early warning signs** to help you watch out for signs of worsening depression or anxiety.
- Find out about how to set up your own regular **review session** to help you put into practice what you have learned.
- Discover how to access other five-areas materials and other useful support resources.

Planning for the future

This section summarises some principles that you may find helpful when it comes to planning how to face the future. It can sometimes be helpful to think of yourself as being on a **journey of recovery**. When you first started working on your problems, it is likely that you had a range of different problems you wished to tackle. During the treatment, it is to be hoped that things have improved in at least some areas since you began your journey down this path.

The following are some questions to help you identify **what** has been helpful for you and what things have helped you move on. Write down your thoughts in the space below each question. What is different now compared with before? What gains have I made? How have I improved in each of the five areas?

(?) In my thinking?

✎

....

....

....

(?) In my feelings and in the physical symptoms I notice?

✎

....

....

....

? In my behaviour and activity levels? What I can and can't do, and whether I respond to things in helpful or unhelpful ways.

✎

....

....

....

? In the practical situations, relationships and practical problems that I face? What practical resources have I discovered in myself and in the support from others around me?

✎

....

....

....

What have I done to make these changes happen?

✎

....

....

....

? In my thinking?

✎

....

....

....

? In my actions?

✎

....

....

....

? What new skills have I gained that I can use to help me continue to improve?

✎

....

....

....

(?) How can I continue to use what I have learned in my everyday life?

....

....

....

(?) What things might get in the way of me doing this? How can I deal with these obstacles? What practical steps can I take?

....

....

....

Try to see whether you can summarise what you have learned as your own **mental fitness plan**. The following example summarises what Paul, who had experienced problems of low mood and stress, has learned on his journey to recovery:

(e.g.) EXAMPLE

Paul's mental fitness plan

- When I begin to feel depressed and anxious, I need to do something about it before it worsens.

- I **can** control my negative thoughts by using the thought workbook.

- Don't withdraw from others when I feel down – they can really help me pick up.

- Avoid drinking too much alcohol – it only makes things worse.

- When I feel overwhelmed by problems, just tackle them one at a time.

To help you create your own mental fitness plan, read the list below. This summarises some key things to do and not do. Tick those that apply to you. This is followed by a further task to help you add any additional things you have learned to create your own plan.

My mental fitness plan

Some things to do	Tick here if this affects your own life, even if only sometimes
Tackle things early if you feel worse/build on your strengths/resources	
Stop, think and reflect on negative thoughts: don't let extreme and unhelpful thinking take over	
Keep doing things that you value – these activities will give you a sense of pleasure and achievement	
Live reasonably healthily in terms of activity, food and sleep – but not obsessively so	
Say no – balance demands you put on yourself – allow space and time for you	
Use relaxation tapes and techniques if you find them helpful, such as anxiety-control training described at our support site www.livinglifetothefull.com	
If you are prescribed an antidepressant medication take it regularly; any changes are best discussed with your own doctor	

Some things not to do	Tick here if this affects your own life, even if only sometimes
Drink too much alcohol	
Let problems build up unaddressed	
Let your thinking spiral out of control	
Avoid things/put things off. Instead, face up to your fears – don't let avoidance take over	
Do things that end up backfiring/worsening things, e.g. taking on too much or setting yourself up to fail	

Additional things I have learned

Now try this for yourself. You can write down as many or as few additional lessons you have learned as you want.

✎

....

....

....

What else have you learned about getting and staying better?

1

2

3

4

5

1

Section 2 **Looking for signs of relapse**

Watch for difficult times

One of the most important things is to watch for difficult times so that you can plan out in advance what to do if you are beginning to feel worse for whatever reason. Sometimes, certain situations make people feel especially bad or seem particularly difficult to cope with. Everyone is different. They could include times such as:

- **Personal losses:** when you feel let down, rejected or abandoned by someone, e.g. after a relationship difficulty or breakdown. Other common losses include bereavement, loss of job and retirement.
- **Setbacks/challenges:** when something important seems to have gone wrong or you have a fear that it will go wrong.
- **Stress:** when you think things are beginning to get out of control.
- **Stopping or reducing antidepressants:** there can be an increased risk of feeling worse for a few weeks or months.

 What are my possible high-risk situations in terms of setbacks?

1

2

3

What do I need to do differently if I encounter these situations?

1

2

3

Watch for early warning signs of slipping back

One helpful approach is to try to watch out for **early signs** that problems such as depression or anxiety are worsening. These often show a pattern that can be watched for. Try to write out a short list of **early warning signs** to watch out for. This may include things like:

- **Situation, relationship and practical problems:** a build-up of problems that begin to feel overwhelming.
- **Altered thinking:** noticing more negative or worrying thoughts that dominate your mind.
- **Altered feelings:** such as feeling down and low or beginning to feel anxious.

- **Altered physical symptoms:** for example, growing tension or restlessness, or a worsening of sleep or appetite.
- **Altered behaviour – reduced or avoided activities:** beginning to withdraw from others or activities (reduced activity) or increasingly avoiding certain situations (e.g. by staying in bed later and later).
- **Altered behaviour – unhelpful reactions to things:** drinking much more alcohol or doing other things that can worsen how you feel.

Sometimes it can help to also talk to others who you know and trust to discover whether they have noticed any other early warning signs. You could also ask them to tell you if they think you are struggling or slipping back. Perhaps you could give them a copy of your fitness plan so they know what to look out for.

The following example summarises how Anne looked back to identify her own early warning signs of recurring depression.

 EXAMPLE

Anne's early warning signs

Anne has identified that her early warning signs are:

- **Situation, relationship and practical problems:** feeling overwhelmed by problems and not acting to overcome them.

- **Altered thinking:** becoming very negative and predicting that things will go badly (negative predictions). Having a very negative view of myself. Overlooking good things that happen (negative mental filter).

- **Altered feelings:** feeling low and weepy, and also feeling very little at all, as though my emotions are becoming numb.

- **Altered physical feelings/symptoms:** feeling very low in energy and finding it difficult to get up in the morning.

- **Altered behaviour:** a tendency to want to withdraw and ask my sister not to visit. Stopping doing things I normally enjoy, such as going for a walk or going to the shops.

In addition, it can be helpful if Anne can identify **one key early warning sign**. This should be a key symptom that she can watch for and that was present quite early on when she became depressed before.

My key early warning sign: 'I am going to watch out for times when I feel really tired – not just a bit tired, but times when I feel exhausted all the time and just want to stay in bed.'

This key early warning sign means: **do something now to tackle how you feel**.

EXAMPLE

Paul's early warning signs

Paul has identified that his early warning signs are:

● **Situation, relationship and practical problems:** beginning to put off handing in work and becoming unassertive in sorting things out. Letting problems go unaddressed.

● **Altered thinking:** mind-reading that others don't like me. Losing confidence. Predicting the worst will happen (catastrophising).

● **Altered feelings:** feeling low and weepy or starting to feel very anxious all the time.

● **Altered physical symptoms:** feeling really tense and jittery.

● **Altered behaviour:** trying to block how I feel by drinking more alcohol than normal. Beginning to avoid things that seem scary.

My key early warning sign: 'I am going to watch out for times when I feel I lose confidence and start mind-reading what others think of me.'

My early warning signs

Now try to create your own list of early warning signs:

Situation, relationship and practical problems:

✎

....

....

....

Altered thinking:

✎

....

....

....

Altered feelings:

✎

....

....

....

Altered physical symptoms:

✎

....

....

....

Altered behaviour:

✎

....

....

....

My **key early warning sign:**

✎

....

....

....

The purpose of creating this early warning list is so that you can plan to make changes at an early stage.

Producing an emergency plan

Imagine you live in a house that has a smoke detector. One day you hear it beeping while you are watching television. What do you do? Do you ignore it and keep watching the television as if there was no problem? Or do you get up, find out whether there is a problem and try to deal with it? In the same way, if you notice any of your **early warning signs**, you need to have planned what you will do in response. This should include making sure you are putting your personal **mental fitness plan** into practice. It may also need to include some other responses if this alone doesn't improve how you feel.

The plan should include involving others:

- Choose to stay in contact with people who support you. Choose not to isolate yourself. Tell others you trust that you are noticing some problems.
- Go and talk to a healthcare practitioner about your problems and discuss whether you need more help. This might include being prescribed an antidepressant or seeing a mental health specialist such as a clinical psychologist, psychiatrist or nurse.

You might also plan to make changes. An **emergency plan** can help you to plan out how to tackle any early warning signs you notice.

The following example shows how Anne decides to react to her early warning signs.

EXAMPLE

Anne's emergency plan

Early warning sign	Emergency plan
Altered thinking: with negative predictions and mind-reading	Identify and challenge extreme and unhelpful thinking
Altered feelings: feeling low and weepy	Do all of the above things, and also go to see my doctor to talk about whether other treatments such as an antidepressant may be useful
Altered physical symptoms: feeling low in energy and worse in the morning	Plan to do more difficult tasks later on in the day; do things at a reasonable pace
Altered behaviour: withdrawing from doing things I like	Create an action plan to do things that give me a sense of pleasure and achievement
Altered behaviour: asking my sister Mary not to visit	Choose to ask Mary over each week for a short period of time

My emergency plan

What is your **emergency plan** in the event of a setback? Try to be very specific about the things you could do. Include your own mental fitness plan as well as any people you could contact to help you.

1

2

3

4

5

If your problems begin to worsen in spite of your plan, go to the professionals. If a fire was beginning to worsen at home in spite of your attempts to tackle it, you would call for professional help. Similarly, if you feel worse in spite of your emergency plan, get in touch with your previous healthcare practitioner or your doctor. They will be able to advise you as to whether other additional approaches such as the use of medication may be helpful.

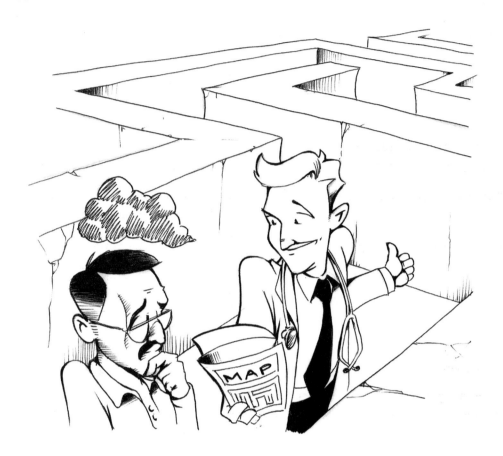

Section 3   **Keeping things going: the concept of a regular review day**

It is important to **continue** using the information and skills that you have learned during the next few months and into the future. One of the advantages of using a workbook such as this is that it allows you to set particular goals and to review how things have gone. You can also **do this yourself** by setting up a **regular review day**.

Developing a regular review day

Get a pen and mark the last day of each month as a review session on your calendar. During this review session, try to spend 30 minutes or so thinking back over the previous month. You can plan to do the review day more frequently if you wish (e.g. fortnightly), but the key point is being able to commit yourself to doing it over the long term.

Use the sheet on the next page to structure your review.

(task)

My review day

Date

✎

....

Since my last review:

What's gone well?

✎

....

....

....

What hasn't gone so well? Am I slipping back? (Review your warning signs list/emergency plan if needed.)

✎

....

....

....

What can I learn from what has happened?

✎

....

....

....

How can I put what has been learned into practice?

✎

....

....

....

My plan for the next few weeks (consider short-, medium- and long-term changes):

What am I going to do?

1

....

....

....

2

....

....

....

3

....

....

....

How will I try to make sure that I carry out my plan?

✎

....

....

When am I going to do it?

✎

....

....

What can prevent this happening? What problems/difficulties could arise, and how can I overcome these? What might sabotage my plan?

✎

....

....

Apply the **questions for effective change** to your plan. Is my planned task one that:

Will be useful for understanding or changing how I am?	Yes ☐	No ☐
Is a specific task, so that I will know when I have done it?	Yes ☐	No ☐
Is realistic, practical and achievable?	Yes ☐	No ☐
Makes clear what I am going to do and when I am going to do it?	Yes ☐	No ☐
Is an activity that won't be easily blocked or prevented by practical problems?	Yes ☐	No ☐
Will help me to learn useful things, even if it doesn't work out perfectly?	Yes ☐	No ☐

Date of my **next review** (do I need to do this more often?)

✎

....

....

....

Write down an **action plan** that you can put into practice over the following week. Try to set specific goals and targets. Plan in some activities that you personally value. These will lead you to have a sense of achievement or pleasure. Plan also to tackle practical problems, avoidance or any unhelpful responses. Choose targets you can achieve. Make changes one step at a time.

The purpose of the review session is to spend a little time to stop, think, reflect and plan how to move forwards.

Finally, remember that you are not alone. Your healthcare practitioner or doctor is there as a resource to work with you and help you move forwards. You can discuss any problems or difficulties with them.

Other resources that offer information and support

 A range of voluntary-sector self-help groups and organisations can offer support and information. The Prodigy NHS website www.prodigy.nhs.uk links to many such organisations and also brings together in one place patient leaflets and resources for a wide range of physical and mental health problems.

Some general information and resources online

Website	Comment
Living Life to the Full: www.livinglifetothefull.com	Free online life-skills course – companion site to these workbooks. Written by Dr Chris Williams. Contains discussion forums and teaching materials supporting the use of the various workbooks in the course. Also includes a download area to print off the key handouts and worksheets used in the various five-areas courses
British Association for Cognitive and Behaviour Therapies (BABCP): www.babcp.com	Lead body for cognitive behaviour therapy in the UK. Provides a range of free leaflets that are updated frequently
Mind: www.mind.org.uk/information/factsheets	Wide range of free-to-read leaflets. Can be read but not printed; also available for purchase
Northumberland self-help materials: www.nnt.nhs.uk/mh/ content.asp?pagename=selfhelp	Excellent series of self-help leaflets addressing a wide range of life skills such as overcoming anger, guilt, shame, low mood, etc.
MoodGYM: http://moodgym.anu.edu.au	Excellent site offering a free online course aimed at preventing depression
Prodigy NHS central patient resource: www.prodigy.nhs.uk	Excellent central one-stop shop

Some books

Chris Williams (2003) *Overcoming Anxiety: A Five Areas Approach*. London: Hodder Arnold. Focusing on generalised anxiety/worry, panic and phobias, obsessive–compulsive disorder (OCD) materials and anxiety in physical health problems.

Chris Williams, Paul Richards and Ingrid Whitton (2002) *I'm Not Supposed to Feel Like This: A Christian Self-help Approach to Depression and Anxiety*. London: Hodder and Stoughton.

Workbook summary

In this workbook you have:
- Summarised what you have learned about getting better.
- Created a mental fitness plan to use in the future.
- Produced a list of your own early warning signs to help you watch out for signs of worsening depression or anxiety.
- Found out about how to use a regular **review session** to help you put into practice what you have learned.
- Discovered how to access other five-areas materials and useful support resources.

Putting into practice what you have learned

You may find it helpful to re-read this and other workbooks on a regular basis. Consider building this reading into your regular review sessions. Discuss this with your doctor or healthcare practitioner.

A request for feedback

An important factor in the development of all the five areas assessment workbooks is that the content is updated on a regular basis based upon feedback from users and practitioners. If there are areas that you find hard to understand or seem poorly written, please let me know and I will try to improve things in future. I regret that I am unable to provide any specific replies or advice on treatment. To provide feedback, please contact us by:
- *Website:* www.livinglifetothefull.com.
- *Email:* feedback@livinglifetothefull.com.
- *Post:* Dr Chris Williams, Psychological Medicine, Gartnavel Royal Hospital, 1055 Great Western Road, Glasgow G12 0XH.

Acknowledgements

I wish to thank all those who have commented upon this workbook, especially Marie Chellingsworth.

My notes

....
....
....
....
....
....
....
....
....
....
....
....
....
....
....
....
....
....
....
....
....
....
....
....
....

My notes

....
....